Swimming on My Wedding Day

Swimming on My Wedding Day

My Cancer Journey through the Seasons

Laura Fitzpatrick-Nager

Foreword and Illustrations by
Paul Fitzpatrick-Nager

iUniverse, Inc.
New York   Lincoln   Shanghai

Swimming on My Wedding Day
My Cancer Journey through the Seasons

Copyright © 2008 by Laura Fitzpatrick-Nager

All rights reserved. No part of this book may be used or reproduced by any means, graphic, electronic, or mechanical, including photocopying, recording, taping or by any information storage retrieval system without the written permission of the publisher except in the case of brief quotations embodied in critical articles and reviews.

iUniverse books may be ordered through booksellers or by contacting:

iUniverse
2021 Pine Lake Road, Suite 100
Lincoln, NE 68512
www.iuniverse.com
1-800-Authors (1-800-288-4677)

Because of the dynamic nature of the Internet, any Web addresses or links contained in this book may have changed since publication and may no longer be valid.

The views expressed in this work are solely those of the author and do not necessarily reflect the views of the publisher, and the publisher hereby disclaims any responsibility for them.

ISBN: 978-0-595-42655-3 (pbk)
ISBN: 978-0-595-86983-1 (ebk)

Printed in the United States of America

For Paul
and
Mom and Dad

*I feel my boots trying to leave the ground, I feel my heart pumping hard.
I want to think again of dangerous and noble things.
I want to be light and frolicsome. I want to be improbable beautiful
and afraid of nothing as though I had wings.*
—Mary Oliver

Contents

Acknowledgments xi
Foreword xv
Prologue xix

Season 1: My Turn 1
    Round One 3
    Surveillance 6
    Round Two 8
    A Second Primary 9
    Breast Sightseeing 11
    My Mastectomy 14
    Memory in the Mirror 16
    Engaging Times 17
    Chemo Sonnets 19
    Bad-Hair Day 21
    Wig Days 22
    With This Ring 24

Season 2: Paul's Turn 27
    Déjà Vu 29
    The Waiting Game—Again 31
    The Art of Sperm Banking 34
    Weary Days 36

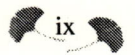

Underground Losses 39
Unwanted Commitments 41
House Hunting 43

Season 3: My Turn—Again 47
Round Three: Recurrence 49
Moving Day 52
The Miracle Jar 55
Morning Poem 60
Where the Wild Things Are 61
Recovery Notes 65
A Letter to My Doctor 68

Season 4: Homecoming 73
A Poem from Paul 75
Ginkgo Day 76
Spa Secrets 80
An Anniversary Letter to Paul 84
My Ovary Party 86
Called to Rise 88
The Face of Healing 90
Blossoms 93

Acknowledgments

There are words that fall short of the magnitude they carry. *Thank you* is one of those phrases. It doesn't convey nearly the depth of what's in my heart, but here goes:

To those friends who have been midwives to this book, and to me, I say thank you, including Letty Russell, Christina Giebisch, Maggie Marshall, Catherine Keyes, Sue Lavoie and my mom, Elaine McNally Fitzpatrick. To my dear friend and tireless editor, Christina Giebisch, I add boundless thanks for keeping me on track up until I hit the send button. To Cindy Boynton, thank you for your editorial help early on in my writing.

To my former boss and mentor, Dr. Patricia Sweeting, of Teachers College, Columbia University: my sincerest appreciation for your encouragement and care while I juggled work and treatment.

To the medical experts whose care I received over the years: Dr. Samuel Bobrow, Dr. Joseph Cardinale, Dr. Thomas Kolb, Dr. Anne Moore and Dr. Kimberly J. Van Zee. You are true healers in the medical profession. To Deb Del Vecchio-Scully, Manager of the Integrative Medicine program at the Father McGivney Center for Cancer Care at St Raphael's Hospital, thank you for the faithful wisdom, practical advice, and insights you've shared with me. In addition, I offer thanks to Leslie Blatt, APRN, and to all my friends in the Life Enhancement support group. Your nurturing voices strengthened my own. To Ellen Swirsky, friend and founder of the Looking Forward program at St Raphael's Hospital, I bow deeply to the inspiration you have given me and many others.

To all of the cancer survivors I interviewed in the initial stages of this book, I say thank you: Marcie Casey, Nancy Bruno, Margo Gross, Barbara Oliver of Y-Me, Jane Bannerman, Debbie Braun, Pat Bullard,

Peg Heitmann, Toni Smith, Carolyn Johns, Jeanne Thomsen, Ruth Ann Lobo, Joan Shrewsbury, Ilse Giebisch, and Celestine Pleasure. Speaking with you helped me to find my own path through the wilderness of the recurrent cancer journey. My listening lessons began in your kitchens and living rooms; you opened a road of hope in me while serving me cups of tea.

To my writing teacher, Natalie Goldberg, and my writing intensive buddies at the Mabel Dodge Luhan House, thank you for teaching me about Taos Mountain, the power of silence, floating down the Rio Grande, and writing practice. To Bob, Jude, and Joanne, I say three Guinnesses and a margarita—*Ten minutes. Go.*

To Janet Weber, many thanks for your spiritual guidance through the dark night and morning light.

To my parents, Richard and Elaine, your unwavering strength, support, and love are an example to me of how not only to live, but to *thrive,* whatever life throws at you. When I didn't think I could go on, you carried me *and* let us move in!

My gratitude also extends to many other family members who kept encouraging me with this project. To my sister, Julie, thank you for your creative genius, sparkling talents, and Julie-love. I also thank my brother, David, who knows how writing can save a life and has his own story to tell someday soon. You have taught me what resiliency is.

To Dennis, Rick, Mary, Christopher, and Dominic, the newest member of our clan, loving thanks for your presence in my life. To my dear cousin, Sheila, thank you for the note-taking and countless hours you spent with us at our medical appointments. To my cousins-in-law, Deb and Julie, thanks for the big love, poetry, and wings. To my mother-in-law, Dora, your Friday night prayers came in handy many times over.

To my Aunt Marion, fellow cancer survivor and friend, your support has been as sweet as the music you make on your violin, many thanks.

And to my dear husband, Paul, who teaches me every day about love, home, and living in the moment no matter how high the watermark might be, *you* have made all the difference.

Poet Li-Young Lee sums it up this way:
There are days we live as if death
were nowhere in the background;
from joy to joy,
from wing to wing,
from blossom to impossible blossom,
to sweet impossible blossom.

Thank you all for walking with me through the seasons.

Foreword

It was Labor Day 1995 when I met Laura in Acadia National Park in Maine. I was on my yearly pilgrimage for rock climbing, beer, and lobster. Laura had arrived with a mutual friend and was one of the *single* women. My chemistry started jumping around the first time we met. I flexed my muscles when she thought I didn't see her looking, tried to get close whenever I could, and went bike riding with her when I could have been climbing. And so the dance began. From the start, I was crazy about her.

Long before we met, I spent a fair amount of time in the mountains. Up high is where I feel most comfortable. There's no malice in nature, even when it's storming—and I especially like a good storm.

One winter, a friend and I were out for a weekend of camping on Mount Chocorua in New Hampshire. We had hiked to the edge of the tree line and dug ourselves in. A storm was coming, and we knew we were in for a rather exciting evening. By 4:30 that afternoon, we'd prepared our camp as best we could, finished setting up, and changed into dry clothes. We were just hunkering down to start dinner when we felt the wind pick up. There is an odd anticipation in this setting—it's wildness in the wilderness, and as much confidence as you might have in your ability to prepare and deal with the circumstances at hand, you can be sure fear will be part of the evening's equation. Apparently, I was in training for bigger things—it makes for a long night on a mountaintop in winter. You can really hear the storm coming ...

Laura showed up on my doorstep one Friday night not long after we had gotten back together. She had driven up to Boston for the weekend. When I opened the door, she was standing there crying. "It's back," she said. "The cancer's back." It was that night, as we held on to each other, that I decided I was here for the long run. I had no idea

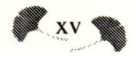

how prepared I was for what was moving in our direction, but I could hear the storm coming.

On Christmas Eve of 1998, I asked Laura to marry me. She had just gone through major surgery a few days before. We were lying in bed, and I remember having this little conversation in my head. *What can I do to help? What can I do? ... What can I do? ... Well, Paulie boy, you're going to ask her to marry you at 'some point' ... so ... why not right now? Let's have something to smile about right now! Wedding ... honeymoon ... look forward ... choose life ... seek joy ... okay ... okay ... do it ... Okay ...* "Laura ..."

And so, I proposed, and she said, "Yes," and we spent the next six months planning a wedding and a honeymoon—all of which Laura will tell you about. I just wanted to give you a little spousal perspective before you went on ...

It's quite an emotional balancing act, this cancer business ... We placed our lives in the hands of others and hoped and prayed they would have *all* the answers, that they would make this *all* go away. From the moment you hear the words, "You have cancer," something shatters inside of you ... Perhaps it's your innocence. We all know we will die someday. Those of us in the cancer club have faced our pending mortality with a rawness that the "philosophy" of dying can't touch. We have been forever changed. There is so much to deal with ... and it is so easy to fall into the darkness that this disease brings with it.

Throughout our last eight years together, Laura has had cancer, I have had cancer, and Laura has had cancer again. We have been harbor to an emotional storm that rages and ebbs, and each time, we have found something to keep us in the world—something to work at. It was good to have a goal, but it would be the process that would take us away from cancer.

I painted and, with help from our family and friends, built our house. Laura went from keeping a journal to becoming a writer. We were going to build our future no matter what the obstacles were. Cancer would not keep us from living. Cancer would not keep us from being happy. Cancer was going to teach us about life ... and about love.

I am so honored to be a part of this story. I've watched it progress from inception to completion—in all its phases. I've watched Laura grow in her craft, develop confidence in her abilities, and move beyond the trauma. It is in Laura's nature to express herself through writing, as it is in her nature to help others who are going through troubled times.

So let's see ... we got married, went to Paris and Provence for a honeymoon, visited Hawaii, built our house, I got to be an artist again, and Laura has written this book.

We have gone through our share of trials and tribulations, but our bottom line has stayed the same—life, love, and the pursuit of happiness together. I've never questioned my decision that Christmas Eve ... and with all the water that's gone under the bridge, I'm still crazy about her.

Paul Fitzpatrick-Nager
August 2007

Prologue

Front and center on our refrigerator is a memorable photo of us on our wedding day. The reception was nearing the finale, and we found ourselves on the edge of something cool and brave in the humid July heat. Paul was whisked off the packed dance floor by several ushers and carried out to the pool area. Splash! Paul was thrown in—Calvin Klein tux and all. I followed the crowds to see Paul floating belly up. Our friend, Steve, quietly asked me, "Care to go for a swim?"

I looked down at my silk satin gown and hesitated. Cathy, my best friend from college, nudged my arm, whispering, "The Laura I know would jump in that pool!"

That was all the encouragement I needed. With our wedding party in tow, Paul and I lined up on the rim of the sparkling pool hand in hand. My bare toes perched on the hot cement ready for liftoff. On the count of three, we jumped for joy. My mother, our minister on that magical day, still hasn't forgiven me for not changing out of my gown first.

This picture of Paul and me floating in our finery often reminds me that I am not alone on this journey called life. It was taken four months after I'd completed chemotherapy for invasive breast cancer. My black, curly hair, too short for a veil, was crowned with garland and lace from my cousin Sheila's wedding. Little did we know on that day that Paul too would be diagnosed with cancer on our first wedding anniversary and then go through intense rounds of chemotherapy similar to my own or that I would be diagnosed with a recurrence of breast cancer shortly after Paul's recovery. Our wedding day, remarkable as it was, could not protect us from the tidal waves life would send us both.

But, just as on that poolside wedding day, we have continued to be surrounded by support on all sides. Friends and family were our lifejackets throughout our newly married life together. Sometimes we'd be rescued by one of their passing lifeboats. On other days, we'd paddle upstream on our own. Despite many days of choppy waters, cancer treatments, and life changes, Paul and I haven't had to travel this uncertain path alone. We are so lucky.

This book of reflections has grown out of my diagnoses and recovery. I've been a journal writer since high school when I began to write down my life in my first blue bound notebook. Seeing my words grow on paper day after day helped me to inch out of this life crisis called cancer. Writing is a healing practice for me. My quest is for a life free of disease—a long life, preferably. Along my healing path, I've found such abundance—especially inner reservoirs of strength I never knew I possessed.

My book is divided into four seasons. Season One contains vignettes of my initial cancer diagnosis and recovery. Similarly, Season Two offers a view of Paul's cancer experience and our life at that specific time. My memory and writing of those early seasons are more a series of snapshots than a flowing narrative—a result of the trauma, I suspect. In Seasons Three and Four, my reflections take on an essay format as I gain perspective on my life and the road I didn't choose but made my own. I've elected to leave the variations in my writing style as a sign of the changes that unfolded within me. Journal entries are included within each season.

When I set out to write this book, it was initially an act of desperation. I needed hope. I needed to know how to live through the recurrent cancer journey. "You didn't create this," said a wise friend, "but you can create your healing." I carry these words of wisdom with me to this day. For me, writing down the bones of my story has helped me carve out the seasons of my recovery.

Originally, my book started as an anthology of hope about other women cancer survivors. I wanted to know their secrets of survivorship. *How did you do it?* I asked. *How did you deal with the fear, find hope, live a day without the burden of it?* With my tape recorder, tapes, yellow legal pad, and fast writing pens packed in my bag, I set out for my interviews. I had a long list of survivors to choose from. There was hope in numbers!

In all, I met with eighteen women between the ages of thirty-two and ninety-two. I'd spend an hour or two with each of them, sipping tea in their kitchens, looking through photo albums in their living rooms, or meeting them at the office they'd returned to after cancer. The youngest, at thirty-two, was pregnant and soon to give birth to a healthy little boy named Jack. And, at ninety-two years old, my friend's great-aunt Jane shared with me her watercolor sketchbooks and paintings of world travels. I also encountered several mothers, a pediatrician, two teachers, a realtor, three grandmothers, several artists, a harpist-minister, an activist, a massage therapist, and many friends. These wise women were my first support group, a lineage of hope I'd become a member of. I recorded their words in hopes of mining a secret for myself. I spent hours hunched over my laptop, transcribing my notes and writing out first impressions.

In the end, I organized their life experiences into a kind of wellness map for myself. I discovered that each person had found a unique way to keep living and embracing her life, despite cancer's ugly intrusion. And in between the lines of their wisdom, my own story grew louder. *Pick me! Pick me!* the voice urged. The gift of their survivor stories helped shape my own circuitous path.

Bearing witness to one another's lives is the greatest gift we can give each other. Here is my story, nurtured through many seasons of hope, loss, lasting gifts, and steadfast love.

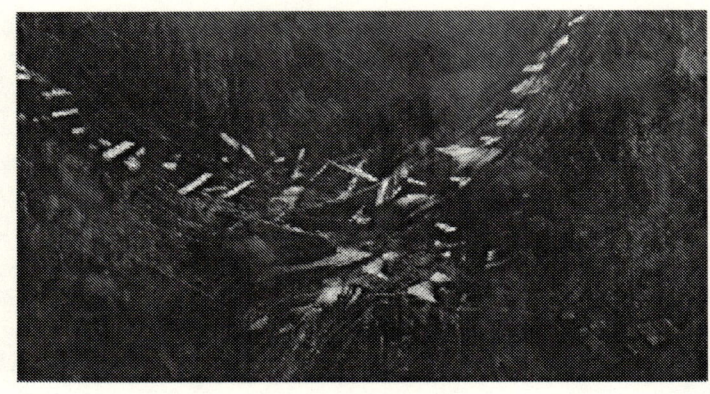

*Hope is the thing with feathers
that perches in the soul
and sings the tune without the words
and never stops at all.*

—Emily Dickinson

Season 1

My Turn

Round One

I'd just blown out thirty-four pink and yellow candles on my chocolate birthday cake when I was diagnosed with the C word. Everyone was shocked that I was so young, had no family history, ate my fruits and veggies, and *seemed* to be so healthy. One day, I was meeting friends for lunch looking très chic in a sunny flowered sundress. The next, I was pushing open the glass revolving doors leading to oncology clinic rooms. Wearing a paper-thin hospital gown, I endured rounds of biopsies. My cancer journey began out of the blue, without a trace of warning.

In my case, the first time the cancer appeared was hard to ignore. I remember the silvery knit shirt I wore one Saturday night on the town. Looking down at my chest as I closed my menu, I noticed faint red stains had soaked through my clothes. My right nipple was bleeding. Years later, I found that shirt balled up in a forgotten box and threw it away, the faint outline of rusty stains still visible.

After two days of watching my breast leak blood slowly like an almost flat tire, I called my doctor. My gynecologist sent me to have a mammogram and wait for results. Statistics were never a strong point for me, even in college. I was told there was a 95 percent chance it was nothing. *Great,* I thought, *what's there to worry about?*

Nothing turned out to be ductal carcinoma in situ—a little breast cancer.

I remember the phone call from the surgeon. Her brisk tone of voice on the other end of the line told me the news was not going to be cheery. "I've got good news and bad news," she said. "What would you like first?"

Like? I would like you to go away, I thought.

"It was breast cancer, but very, very tiny," she continued, "so tiny you should just go on with your life, no treatment needed. We'll just do a lumpectomy and watch you closely," my doctor advised.

Without delay, I had a lumpectomy of my right breast. Peeking under the small bandage after surgery, I was relieved to see that the scars were barely visible, but everything had changed. In my journal, I wrote down my churning fears:

> *I'm not invincible anymore. I'd never thought of my body as anything but healthy. I am in good shape, aren't I? You can't tell I have cancer by looking at me. I often jog the three-mile reservoir in Central Park, play tennis. I even ran the Boston Marathon in college.*
>
> *Where did the cancer cells come from? Did they wiggle up the rusted pipes of my 1940s brick apartment building into my pasta water? Or burrow in my body with the stress of subway riding and teaching developmentally challenged teenagers housed in an asbestos heap of a school building? Maybe it was the runoff from the cranberry bogs on Cape Cod where I spent my summers ever since I was seven years old.*
>
> —*May 1997*

Cancer was not a word I knew anything about. No one in my family circle had ever had breast cancer. I didn't know anyone who did. In my family, we had other things like depression, diabetes, and death from being old with emphysema. With cold sweats and heart pounding, questions bubbled up from my gut and onto the page one morning:

> *What do I do now? Should I get a second opinion? Where do I find the best treatment? Am I going to die? I'm scared to even see that last sentence in black and white.*
>
> —*May 1997*

My questions didn't have quick answers. After reading all of the Dr. Love Breast books my mom and I could get our hands on, we decided to pursue a second opinion. In the scheme of things, this initial diagnosis and recommendation to "just go on with your life" sounded pretty good, but we needed to make sure there were no lingering cells wandering around. We had a follow-up plan. I felt in control.

Since I was living in Manhattan at the time, we selected Memorial Sloan-Kettering, a renowned medical center, for my second opinion. Their motto, "the best cancer care anywhere," was reassuring. My apartment on the Upper East Side was near the hospital. I can recall how at that moment, my reference point was forever altered. My inner compass shifted with my cancer diagnosis. When I walked out of my apartment most mornings, I faced not only my neighborhood bagel shop and a brick Episcopal church but was suddenly aware of the hospital a few blocks away. I'd never even paid attention to it before.

After a lengthy consultation with my new medical team, a second procedure of the same area of my breast was recommended by the physicians, just to ensure all the diseased tissue had been removed. More tissue was sampled to ensure the area was clean.

> *I no longer have to worry about a clean apartment but being clean in my body. Weird, the language of cancer: Malignant, tumor, dirty margins. I'm collecting upbeat words to balance out the scary ones: wellness, healing, healthy tissue.*
> *—June 1997*

I now had a breast surgeon and an oncology consultant as my medical team. I was back at work again after several days, stiff and shaken from the turn of events in my life. "Go on with your life" was the message I heard for the second time. So I did and felt reassured by the additional reinforcing news. Outwardly, I looked fine as I walked into classrooms to see my students, but my head was swimming. Everyone I knew had a different opinion about what I should do next to protect myself from cancer. I received books on organic living, shark cartilage, and raw macrobiotic cooking as antidotes to cancer. I considered throwing away all of my cooking pots and buying enamel. Some suggestions I kept; others I tossed—like the recipe for coffee enemas. I preferred a tall, decaf, light Starbucks *over the counter*, thank you very much.

Surveillance

For the next year, I was followed by my new medical team every three months. This was to ensure my getting safely out of the woods. *Surveillance* conjured up images for me of searchlights, prisoners marching outside on cold afternoons, and confessions in the dark. For a cancer patient, surveillance means being checked very closely *forever*. My oncologist told me we needed to keep the flashlight on my cells to prevent further invasion.

Mom and I affectionately called my new breast surgeon "the Flying Nun" as she resembled Sally Fields and always seemed on top of the current research. I trusted her. She listened to my concerns and never took anything I said lightly during my checkups—a key detail when you're entrusting your life (and breast) to someone with a knife. "Whatever decisions you make," she told me during one visit, "always choose the most aggressive thing you can do."

After round one, I was now in the high-risk category, despite my lack of family history. This meant that my mom and sister Julie, eighteen at the time, were now high risk as well. Years later, I realized that this is yet another burden the person with cancer carries. The whole family is affected. It's a wake-up call for everyone.

My checkups were in a commercial building of offices and condos near the hospital. An elevator took me down two floors to a busy waiting room. This pink and white hushed underground place felt miles away from the reality of street level. It was surreal. The room was filled with dozens of people all hanging on as best they could to those they loved. Illness had changed the course of everyone's life here.

These checkup trips up and down the elevator are sobering. It's with a club of riders I hadn't asked to

belong to. In the waiting room, there are women talking in whispers to their husbands, others reading the Times *quietly by themselves, and still others sitting red-eyed in front of the receptionist. There are smartly dressed executives with trendy briefcases and grandmotherly types clutching their purses and tissues. I am so young compared to the rest of this crowd.*
—*September 1997*

It was hard to tell by looking who had cancer and who didn't. I'd walk over to the mini-fridge fully stocked for patients in waiting, grab a water bottle and graham crackers, and wait for my number. When my name was finally called, I'd enter the inner sanctum, remove my work clothes, and don the lavender garment of a patient. Shivering in my gown, my heart thawed when I heard the comforting words I longed for: "You look good. See you next time!" Phew. I slowly exhaled and rode the elevator up to street level, feeling semi-normal again.

I learned not to go alone to these appointments. Not only was there safety in numbers but the element of surprise (from hearing "You have more cancer," for example) was eased with extra support and another set—or two—of ears. Mom usually drove into New York City from Connecticut for my medical appointments and joined my cousin Sheila, who jumped on many a cross-town bus just to sit beside me and take notes. Whenever the word *cancer* was brought up, there was an uncontrollable buzzing in my ear. So far, I'd been lucky.

* * *

During this extended period of surveillance, Paul entered my life. He was an artist with a mischievous twinkle in his brown eyes. "I know the secret of life," he told me as we biked up Cadillac Mountain on Mount Desert Island. We dated on and off for a while. Little did I know that our first encounter in those pine-needled woods of Maine would lead to something more. Three years later, we married. My body seemed to be falling apart, but my heart was becoming whole.

Round Two

While my romance with Paul began and then later blossomed, I continued my breast checkups for over a year. Then, as an added precaution, I was referred for regular sonograms. My young, *perky* breasts, my physician told me, would show up clearer under ultrasound. My first visit to the radiologist changed my life again for the second time.

Slathering clear, cool jelly all over my chest, the radiologist pressed down on each breast with his wand, telling me that this kind of equipment was being tested on fighter planes for military surveillance. That was reassuring in an odd way until his wand stopped over several spots, like a jet hovering over a war zone. Suspicious black holes showed up on his computer screen. "Don't move!" he shouted as he drove a small needle into my breast to sample some tissue. How could I move? I wondered. I couldn't breathe. No one was with me this time. I was *supposed* to breeze in and out of this appointment on my lunch break. I never made it back to my new eight week old position at Columbia University that day.

A Second Primary

The results of the sonogram that November afternoon showed two tumors in the same breast. These mysterious tumors were deep and had never shown up on any mammogram or during the initial lumpectomies I had had the year before. The fighter plane sonogram was worth the trouble if it saved my life. It did. The cancer cells had infiltrated my breast, so I was scheduled for a mastectomy just before Christmas. The rollercoaster was moving fast. I kept track of this latest news in my well-used journal:

> *The choices I have to make now are overwhelming. I'm not eating or sleeping. There's no time. I called a teacher I work with who battled cancer and asked her about her oncologist. I stopped short of asking her what I should do about my new job. The phone is ringing off the hook. I'm talking as fast as I can.*
> *—November 1998*

Ultimately, the treatment choices were up to me. My parents, Paul, and my friends had opinions, but the decisions were mine to live with. Since the beginning of my breast cancer sojourn, I'd been proactive about my medical care. Putting together my own medical team, interviewing a surgeon, and getting second opinions was a full-time job. There should be secretaries for this sort of thing; someone who would spend endless hours on the phone with the insurance company for me. There were days I wished I could take a day off from all of this and go back to my former life, but there was no going back, in spite of how much I wanted to.

Friends of mine had *drycleaners* and *pediatricians* they visited. Here I was thrown into a parallel universe deciding who my breast surgeon and plastic surgeon would be. My cousin had just given birth to a little boy named Ian. I worried that I was giving birth to cancer. Terrified, I didn't know how to handle what was going on inside my own body. Paul would hold me at night and say over and over again how he loved me, how there was hope in choosing life, how this detour was just a part of our life together. Decision-making, overwhelming medical terms, and choices haunted my dreams.

> *Today, my mind's on plastic surgery. Will I wake up after my mastectomy and want something there? What kind of reconstruction is the best for me? Transflap? Implant? One breast, two breasts, no breast?*
> —*December 1998*

Breast Sightseeing

Without question, I decided on a new breast. I wanted to wake up with something already there and in place. Both the mastectomy and initial phase of reconstruction would happen in the operating room on the day of my surgery. Those details I couldn't dwell on too much or I'd hyperventilate. At the suggestion of my newly selected plastic surgeon, I arranged to go breast sightseeing with women who agreed to meet with me and show me their breasts. Lord knows, a picture just wouldn't compare to the real thing.

At my first stop, a petite, matter-of-fact businesswoman named Emily met me at the door of her stylish Upper East Side studio. Standing in her hallway, I was surrounded by Ralph Lauren décor and mahogany paneling. Emily was forty and described how her saline implants now felt after her double mastectomy three years prior to my visit. That was another decision, I thought, panicking. *Do I hold onto one breast or minimize my future risk and cut them both out of my life?*

Emily and I talked at her kitchen table about her recovery and my own upcoming surgery. She said that she only had a few minutes, so time was limited. She was a New Yorker after all, so the clock was ticking and the chitchat short. With little fanfare, Emily lifted her shirt. I stared at her symmetrical, round mounds. I even *copped a feel* putting my palms on her smooth, spongy breasts. They felt like cool, small melons, but they were definitely breasts—*and* they matched. Thanking her with a hug, I reentered the lobby and waited for the elevator. *That was definitely the strangest encounter I've ever had,* I thought.

My second outing was to meet Andrea. "C'mon over," she said over the phone. "My new breast looks wonderful!" I loved her magnetic personality and how upbeat she was. In the next breath, she blurted out her other news. "Two weeks after my last chemo treatment," she exclaimed, "I flew to China to pick up my adopted daughter!" I was speechless. Andrea's story of hope reminded me there was a life beyond cancer—and that fake breasts *are* very real.

A third breast encounter happened over lunch with my friend Cathy. We were about to leave her law office for a quick bite when I was introduced to her colleague. "Do you want to see any more breasts? Denise has two new ones ..." she told me.

I blushed a deep red, cleared my throat, and said, "Sure." Forget lunch. The next thing I knew, we were ushered into a windowless conference room. Locking the door, Denise began unbuttoning her pin-striped blouse as I studied the tiled floor and asked her questions. "Ta da!" she announced as I looked up into two bouncy, generous breasts. *Wow*. Denise proudly arched her shoulders back. Her implants resembled shapely cantaloupes, more like waxed fruit than skin, and without nipples. *But sexy*, I thought, *especially combined with her attitude*. "One more surgery to go." She nodded. I mumbled a compliment and thanked her. I strolled out into the sunshine still hoping for a grilled cheese sandwich. I'd made up my mind. Immediate reconstruction was the way to go and one thing was clear: My reconstructed breast would be a new creature all its own.

Meeting other women survivors who went on with their lives (and with their new breasts) helped me to imagine my body beyond cancer. Years later, I've lifted my shirt too for the newly diagnosed, grateful for the chance to help another woman as I was helped. Being able to share my healing body with another woman has showed me how far I've traveled. Although it doesn't diminish how harrowing an event it is to lose one's breast, it can lessen the fear of the unknown just a little.

Christmas lights were all over Manhattan by now, but I had more weighty concerns on my mind. Nobody knew me as I wandered through Macy's. I resembled other female shoppers while browsing in the intimates section, but loneliness covered me. The crooning of Bing Crosby hung in the air. While shoppers filled their baskets with bright-red sweaters and colorful ornaments, I bought flowered pajamas and matching slippers for my upcoming hospital stay. A friend told me to pack for the hospital with comfort in mind. A few days before, I'd received a surprise gift in the mail: a green plush bathrobe with a heart pin on the lapel from a friend named Grace. As a patient herself, it was so touching that she knew exactly what I needed. In my journal that night, I wrote:

> *My fears are never far away. My greatest fear at this moment is of the anesthesia, that tube down my throat, waking up halfway through, waking up in my hospital room with one less body part. Have I said good-bye to it? How do I do that? Walking into the OR will be just the beginning—no turning back, no running away. God help me. The definition of courage: walking towards the knife.*
> —December 1998

My Mastectomy

In packing for my mastectomy, I made another list and stopped at the pharmacy for toiletries. Would I even *want* to brush my teeth? I wondered. But I stuffed the toothpaste into my small suitcase once I returned home. The doorbell rang, and I rushed down the stairs to meet my folks. They were staying with us for a few days. At the drop of a hat, any time of day or night, they would come.

It was now two weeks before Christmas and the eve of my operation. Keeping busy, Paul and my dad stood on each end of our faded pull-out couch, and decorated our windows with sparkling white lights. It took them hours to adorn the little Brooklyn blue spruce Paul and I had purchased the day before. In the meantime, Mom helped me pack a branch from our tree in my overnight bag—a sweet reminder of these precious moments together. I was loved no matter what happened tomorrow.

* * *

> *I'm home from the hospital. It was brutal. They took away my breast, twenty-six lymph nodes, and a chunk of extra tissue. I remember coming back from the OR to the recovery room. I was in the twilight zone, but I felt the gurney bump into a corner. More stabbing pain. I woke up later unable to move. Paul went to the nurses' station to complain as the morphine drip wasn't working right ... The longest forty-eight hours of my life. Thank God I'm home. My folks leave tomorrow. Poor Paul. He wakes up every four hours to give me the meds so I don't fall behind on the pain game.*
> —December 1998

Those initial days of recovery passed in a groggy haze. I remember being home, propped up by pillows in our bed, watching the afternoon sun filter through a lace curtain. There was a shadowy scrim between me and everyone else. Mom was rubbing my legs with peppermint lotion and bringing me lemon tea. I couldn't turn over because of the sharp needles running up and down my right side. There was a bandaged mound where my breast used to be. I touched it gently and felt the small drainage tubes coming out of my underarm. I shuffled around the apartment in slippers like an old woman.

> *I know I'm getting stronger, but I feel so vulnerable to the pain. Everything aches. New sensations have begun, pulling from the drains and a weird tingling vibrates up my arm. Even my fingertips are numb. It's like my body is settling after the volcano has hit. Every few hours, I have to "strip" the drains and move the fluid through. Luckily, no infection. No news yet on the lymph nodes they took out. But the cancer is out of me.*
> —December 1998

I was overwhelmed by the outpouring of love and support that came our way. The phone rang off the hook with kind messages left by relatives, friends, and students. Our dining room table was covered in flowers. Soothing meditation tapes and CDs came in bright packages sent to me by friends. Our refrigerator was stuffed with lasagna and other comfort foods. We were well taken care of. These gifts were all grace notes that eased our struggle. After five days, I began to feel human again.

> *A bouquet of Hawaiian orchids arrived from Aunt Marion and Uncle Aaron today. Yesterday, a huge blue vase of spring flowers arrived from David. "It's just wildness," Paul said over dinner. I put on lipstick, and we took a walk around the block.*
>
> *I crave normalcy.*
> —December 1998

Memory in the Mirror

I remember the misshapen figure in the bathroom mirror looking back at me. Her big, brown eyes were wide, afraid to look down just yet. *I can do this,* I thought. *I'm still me.* I lifted the bandages a little at a time.

Mom waited on the other side of the door. I could hear her breathing. "Want me to come in?" she asked gently.

"No," I whispered. *Tug,* I winced. Just a little more, *tug,* the tape caught on my skin. *Ouch.* Slowly, one white cotton bandage after another fell into the sink. I raised my head to face the mirror. A swollen, bruised eye, not a breast, peered at me, the lid puffy and exposed. *Oh,* I cried warm tears. I saw a red fault line where my nipple used to be. Mom opened the door and pulled me close.

"It's time to grieve," she said and held me in her arms.

> *The drains came out today. I touched the mottled skin, traced the scar over my breast. There's sensation but it's not anything I've felt before, a numb, faraway feeling. I'll start being inflated with air to stretch my skin for the implant in a few weeks. I can't imagine how I'll look wearing a spare tire on my chest. More tears. Am I more or less of a woman now?*
> —December 1998

Engaging Times

It was the best of times and the worst of times. I recovered in Connecticut at my parents' house over the holiday. We'd learned that the lymph nodes they removed during the mastectomy were clear. Finally, we had good medical news to celebrate. I was set to have chemotherapy once my body healed.

On Christmas Eve, Paul and I were lying in bed talking about how much better I felt. Eight days had passed since the mastectomy; it seemed a lifetime ago. I could sit up and dress myself more easily now but still couldn't raise my arm past my elbow. Suddenly, Paul was on his knees asking me a question, "Will you marry me?" he said softly.

Yes, yes, yes ...

We kept our engagement a secret until New Year's Day. After counting the months on a calendar, we decided to get married the following July on Cape Cod, six months after my mastectomy. Why wait? I hoped my hair would be grown in by then. Would I have enough hair for a veil? Having our marriage day as a goal to reach was truly the light at the end of a long, wintry tunnel.

> *We talked to Deb and Julie today. Julie's designing our rings and ordering some diamond samples. Cool! "What kind of diamond do you want?" she asked me. I have no idea, but I do want a wave motif, something that speaks to the vastness of love, like the ocean, and our riding the waves together.*
>
> *—January 1999*

Planning a wedding in the midst of chemotherapy certainly softened the blow of my treatment. I recommend it as a coping tool. Once the holiday season ended, I began receiving chemotherapy—four rounds every three weeks as long as my body could handle it. We aimed for the most aggressive kind. There wouldn't be a hair on my body left standing—or a cancer cell.

Chemo Sonnets

The rollercoaster of life, love, and cancer continued into the New Year. I was engaged. My scars were healing, and I'd started chemotherapy. Once the semester resumed, I continued to work part-time at Columbia too. All of this happened in a matter of weeks.

> *When I entered the subway today, I stopped to stock up on wedding magazines, my new passion. Finding a dress I like takes my mind off of my next chemo appt. I'm flipping pages like a normal person.*
> —*January 1999*

Our wedding plans became real on the chemo ward. Mom, my sister Julie, and cousin Sheila were my sweet ladies-in-waiting. Luckily, there was a VCR (pre-DVD days) positioned right next to my vinyl recliner. I popped in band videos while a nurse searched for a worthy vein. How much could we spend? Would the band be too loud for the space? Would the jazz trio play the range of music we wanted? These were the pressing questions that filled our hours in the pink room at the Strand Breast Center in Manhattan.

On one treatment day, my sister, Julie, was filled with Shakespeare. She was on her way to an audition for acting school. "Let not the marriage of true minds admit impediments …" she intoned, "even to the edge of doom." The three other patients and my family and I were stunned at her elegant voice. The poignancy of hearing these words spoken from the heart hushed everyone in the room. I knew what Shakespeare meant. But then, as my maid-of-honor-to-be rushed to pick up her bag, Julie smiled again and promptly passed out on the floor at the sight of her sister's IV line. Drama followed us everywhere. I wrote later that night:

> *I'm so nauseous. I can't seem to read for longer than a couple of pages. I don't have the focus or the stomach for it. To keep myself from throwing up, I walk around the dining room table, keeping my legs (and mind) busy. Paul runs out to the store at 10:00 PM to find egg noodles and ketchup, eager for something to do. He also brings back chocolate ice cream. Eating helps. I lick the bowl and start pacing again.*
> —*February 1999*

Bad-Hair Day

As predicted, my hair came out in clumps and handfuls onto my silk pillowcase. Time passed slowly after chemo days. I'd schedule a treatment for Fridays and have the weekend to recover. I'd usually be back to work by Tuesday.

On the way to my second chemotherapy appointment, we stopped at the hair salon for my head shave. I'd gotten up my courage and called my hairstylist a few days before to warn her. Sitting in a private room in the back of the salon, I watched in the mirror as my brown waves fell to the floor. My mother stood behind me like the guardian angel she was. Her face darkened as my head was shorn. Half an hour later, I walked out of the shop onto Fifty-seventh Street, feeling like a punk rocker from the Village with my big, dangling earrings and bare scalp. I felt powerful for the first time in a long while. In my journal, I tried to make sense of this day.

> *My scalp is round and soft to my touch. Little wisps of my hair are still falling out. I kind of like the new do. My head is freezing though. Will I lose my eyebrows and look like the Mona Lisa? My whole body is shedding; a giant Nair factory has rolled over me. My body looks eleven years old again. I feel eighty.*
> *—February 1999*

Wig Days

Many survivors of chemotherapy told me they wore their wigs all the time. I, on the other hand, only wore mine to work. I didn't want to scare anybody out there in the larger world. As heavy as a raccoon hat, my wig's matted fur scratched my scalp like sandpaper. At home, I went au naturel, and Paul often rubbed my head saying, "This is soooo cool." Not to me, it wasn't. A head shave was one thing, but I'd lost my hair *everywhere*. I stared at my bald, prepubescent body in the shower not recognizing myself. I still had eyebrows but that was IT!

The men in my family shaved their heads in solidarity. Paul shaved his goatee and my dad, his graying head. These gestures of love were incredible to me. Paul told me how lost and vulnerable he felt with his beard gone. Dad told me stories of fellow board members at meetings who stared at him strangely and asked if he was sick too. Both Paul and my dad persevered through their own discomfort to walk this journey with me. That was love.

Deep down, with the wig, I felt shielded, protected from the sidelong glances of strangers and students. With wig in hand, I'd gather up my strength for a day's work at the university clinic. It shored up my resolve to treat the day as another ordinary business day with lots of multi-tasking and supervisory meetings with students. Underneath it all, I wanted to pretend my life was going on as usual, that I could handle my job—like superwoman.

> *I gave a workshop to new teachers yesterday with Kathy. I went into the bathroom at lunch and caught a glimpse of myself in the mirror. Yikes! My wig was halfway off my head. Who do I think I'm kidding?*

> *I'm a character on* Saturday Night Live. *So much for vanity.*
> —March 1999

It was hard. A colleague in the next office was growing larger by the day with her first pregnancy and sharing her milk crackers with me as I battled nausea of a different sort. Jane, an assistant, would moan frequently about her recent separation from her husband, seemingly unaware of my own life crisis. Work gave me a sense of purpose, but it also reminded me about how painfully different my life was from my peers. They'd cheer me on by reminding me how few treatments I had left. "Only two more to go, good for you," they'd say. *Do they have any idea how I dread going back into Dr. M.'s office?*

I finished my chemotherapy treatments on schedule. I'd done it. My white blood cell counts were perilously low, but I was finished. I bought a new ivory journal and subscribed to *Bride* magazine.

> *This frightening phase of my life is over. My hair's not growing in fast enough, but I can handle this worry. Sheila gave me her wedding veil today, and we celebrated the end of my treatment with towering hot fudge sundaes. I'm on a sugar high, and I'm alive!*
> —March 1999

Days later, we resumed planning our wedding ceremony with my mother, poring over church details, flower choices, and prayers. I was thrilled that pink and blue hydrangeas would be in season and spectacular that summer. Paul insisted on daisies, his favorite flower. I loved that he cared about the flowers. Only late at night did my loneliness and fear of the future rise up in waves. I hoped for children and a life after this wig—if I was lucky.

With This Ring

Our wedding day lives in my memory as one of the most joyous days of my whole life. At thirty-seven years of age, I'd found my true love, beaten cancer, and lived to tell about it. To us, this day was a day of celebration and gratitude, with all of our favorite people under one sacred roof.

On that hot July morning, my mom, a congregational minister, led our interfaith ceremony. We'd created a Christian and Jewish ritual to reflect both of our histories. We gathered under a wooden chuppah that Paul built for our wedding day. It was the first home he would build for us. In the Jewish faith, the chuppah is a symbol of hospitality, home-making, and relationship. Open on all four sides, this shelter welcomes guests and is meant to be a reminder that our marriage might also be blessed with as many children as there were stars in the heavens. Little did we know then that our dream for children would be particularly challenging—and elude us altogether down the road.

Amidst prayer, poetry, and song, we pledged our lives together repeating our vows: *Your dreams are my dreams, and your love is my blessing.* My mother led us through prayers from both the Irish and Hebrew traditions. She guided us through the ceremony with a gentle hand, strong voice, and proud smile. "Mazeltov!" shouted our family and friends as Paul stepped on the glass under the chuppah. Our new life together began with bells ringing as we walked down the aisle into the steamy sunshine.

Once outside on the lawn, we waited for our guests to flow out of the church. Each held a small pyramid containing a Swallowtail butterfly. These boxes had arrived by the truckload a few days before. On the count of three, we all released them. *Hurrah!* Our joy surrounded us in a cloud of fluttering tuxedo wings.

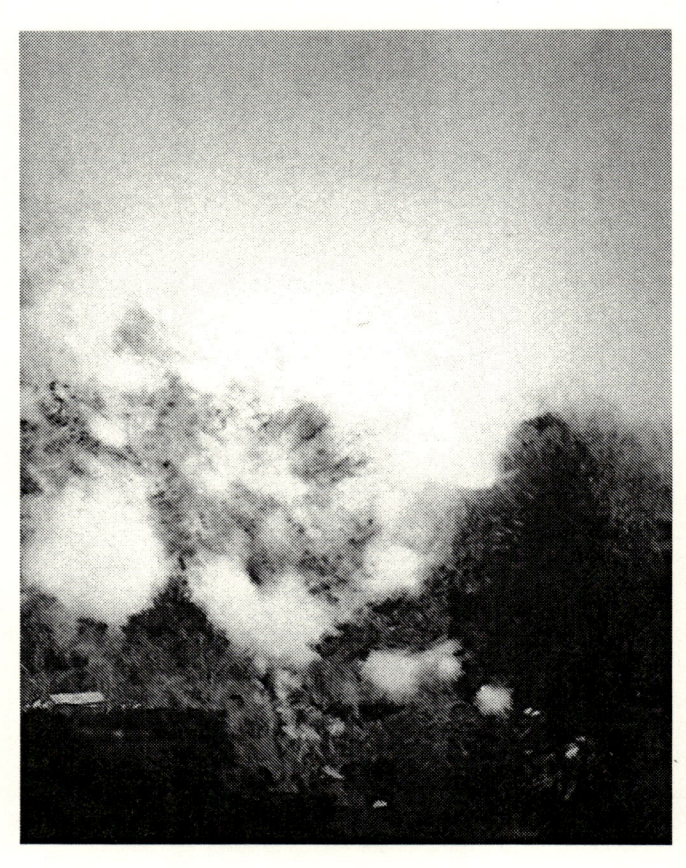

I've found it shelter to speak to you.
—Emily Dickinson

Season 2
Paul's Turn

Déjà Vu

It was New Year's Eve. Friends let us use their chalet in the White Mountains of New Hampshire for the weekend. It was our first married millennium. No one else was invited. We snuck into Tom and Haydie's round hot tub on the front porch and steamed in the frozen air. Shivering, we ran buck naked into the house, dropping borrowed terry-cloth robes in the doorway. It was a peaceful, snowy night, a night of quiet homemade fireworks and chocolate brownies.

> *I'm so happy we've this winter hideaway to ourselves. We watched the world celebrate this new turn of the century on TV last night. I'm a little worried about Paul. His color's not good, and he seems tired for no apparent reason. This morning, I walked through the woods by myself while he lay on the couch.*
> —*January 2000*

Over the next few months, Paul's symptoms worsened. He broke out in cold sweats and shivers, complained of an upset stomach, and was exhausted all the time. Lumps in his groin grew and were tender to the touch, little marbles under the skin. Our general practitioner sent Paul for more tests and then to see an infectious disease guy. Paul had another blood test to rule out Lyme disease. Weeks passed with no real answers. Then, just before our first anniversary, Paul had surgery to remove the pebble-sized nodes.

I sat alone in a dingy waiting room at Cornell Medical Center. I stared at walls the color of pond water. Numb, except for the twitching in my stomach, I watched a nurse wheel Paul through the clinic doors and waved, giving him one more brave smile. Paul's surgeon said I'd have to wait for a couple of hours while they did a "routine exploratory." It felt like we were just a number.

Walking stiffly to the cafeteria, I stood in line to buy an apple and a bowl of cereal for breakfast. I couldn't see the dollars in my wallet through my tears. Someone tapped me on the shoulder, and I turned around to see my Dad standing there. "You came!" I cried as he hugged me. Thank God for my dad. He has always known when to show up and share the load—Always.

The Waiting Game—Again

Our lives changed again in a flash. We were told to wait ten days for the results but not to worry, "it was probably nothing." I tried to ignore the aching familiarity of those words. In the meantime, it was July 24, our first anniversary. Paul moved in slow motion after his biopsy, but we drove up to the Berkshires in Western Massachusetts for a fresh-air weekend away from the hospital. We spent hours poring over our wedding photos. *My hair has grown in so curly since then*, I wrote later that day. The attic room we stayed in at a bed-and-breakfast was yellow and quaint but with the faintest smell of mildew. We rowed onto a placid lake in a wooden canoe and lay in the sun, our oars dipped lazily in the water. I opened a small anniversary package from Paul. He placed a beautiful gold watch on my wrist. We imagined moving to these New England woods in a few years. Was this where we belonged?

Ten long days passed. We drove on another weekend to Cape Cod. *No news was good news* we decided as the sun slipped over the horizon on Bay View Beach. This cape beach was my childhood home and a respite from our unrelenting worries. Finding hermit crabs and stranded starfish, we waded into the chilly salt water up to our kneecaps. I had twenty-seven days off from work, but who was counting? My skin tingled in the heat as I stretched my healing body in the sand next to Paul's sleeping form. Our summer vacation began.

Then, on day two of our vacation, we received the phone call. "It's malignant," said the no-name surgeon on the other end of the line. I heard the feared words. A growl erupted from a deep, primal place in me, up from my belly. I heard Paul's intake of breath on the other end of the line. "Don't leave me," I cried as I wrapped my arms around him. Paul froze and disappeared onto the back porch.

> *Non-Hodgkin's lymphoma has twenty-nine different types. It's a maze of cell division gone awry in the body's lymphatic immune system. Looks like Paul has the aggressive T-cell type, which, in the scheme of cancer things, means "excellent prognosis" and "curable." Hopeful words we cling to like a lifeboat at sea. Paul focused on this note of optimism today. I, on the other hand, am a bruised ball of anger. How could this happen to us? It's a cruel joke. Have you ever met a couple of newlyweds with their own oncologists?*
> —August 1999

We reentered the hauntingly familiar doors of oncology and medical jargon. This time it was *Paul's* hospital, just a few blocks from the pink offices where I had had my own treatment fifteen months earlier. The clinic building resembled an abandoned hospital unit from the 1950s. Our shoes echoed a hollow sound on black-and-white linoleum-tiled floors. I saw faded green everywhere.

Paul's physician came highly recommended as the director of the Lymphoma Center. My only problem with him was that he looked like my twelve-year-old cousin. Did he know absolutely *everything* there was to know to cure my Paul? Dr. Oh-So-Young was in high demand. We waited two to three hours each visit to meet with him. Hospital time was never *on time*. Meanwhile, the taxi horns and sirens on the street reminded me that everyone else's life was going on somewhere else but that ours had come to a complete standstill. Sanity for me became a seat next to the window and a pile of *Country Living* and *Oprah* magazines.

The ground was just beginning to feel solid under my feet after my mastectomy, I wrote in the pocket journal I kept in my purse. I felt betrayed. I read an American Cancer Society brochure that said one out of three people will get cancer. We'd smashed that statistic, hadn't we?

Unlike me, Paul, with his Zen nature, was calm, taking the news as a "minor setback on our journey together." At least that's what he said to make me feel better. Paul joked with friends about his upcoming hairdo and the *silver lining* of having extra time to paint while recovering from treatment. But for me, there was nothing to laugh about.

My bouts of anger disturbed me. They erupted like volcanic ash from a well of grief. That cancer should return to our life again and so soon was unthinkable. I'd harbored the unspoken notion that only one person per family got cancer. I believed they served as a lightning rod to protect the others. I could not imagine watching Paul go through chemotherapy knowing what I knew.

> *So much seems to be coming up for me. It's almost as though I'm going through it all over again. The fear is back, and with it comes a loneliness so deep I can't even speak of it to Paul. He seems so surprised by the depth of my anger. We're in different places with this. Am I crazy?*
>
> *—September 2000*

The Art of Sperm Banking

Among the possible side effects of Paul's approaching treatment was infertility. That side effect was one I'd worried about too during my own chemotherapy. But fortunately, my periods had recently returned along with my strength.

One afternoon, I found Paul surfing the Internet for information on what might happen as a result of his cancer treatment. He was feeling low about the possibility of not having a child the old-fashioned way. Dr. Oh-Too-Young reassured us that there were other ways. Thus, we began our entry into the world of banking—sperm banking, that is.

The language was peculiarly the same as in the financial sphere. One opened an account and made deposits and withdrawals just like at the Bank of America. The only challenge was finding a bank we liked—and trusted. After all, our future progeny would be spending some time there, at least a year or so. Tuition costs, we called them. My mom offered to give us money towards boarding school. We teased her about how expensive grandkids were these days.

I remember opening the thick Manhattan phone book. After all, I couldn't exactly hail a yellow cab and say, "Drop me at the nearest sperm bank." So, instead, we let our fingers do the walking in the Yellow Pages. Two facilities were listed. Since I didn't want to be seen walking into the sperm bank near my office, we chose the second bank, a nondescript but, most important, tidy-looking brownstone in downtown Manhattan.

The sperm technician with the Russian accent suggested we make at least five deposits. Paul grimaced. We'd become adept at saying the word *sperm* out loud to the teller and each other without turning a dark shade of pink. The *room*, however, was a different story. It contained a leather armchair, mood lighting, and a girlie poster—utterly pornographic. My mind wandered as I remembered the space:

> *If this cubicle had been designed with women in mind, it would have been decorated in a warm, shabby chic style with a rose chintz overstuffed chair, glowing candles, and a fluted lamp. Perhaps with an antique night table and the scent of lilacs ...*
> —*September 2000*

For Paul, this was one experience he didn't joke about. After that introductory visit, he asked me to wait at the corner deli for him. So I found a round table near the window and munched on a toasted sesame bagel with jelly while I wrote in my journal. In about twenty minutes, Paul would join me for a cup of coffee, pale and sullen. Mission accomplished.

Weary Days

Chemotherapy also took its toll on Paul. I remember when his tongue was so swollen in his mouth he couldn't talk or eat breakfast. These were symptoms I hadn't experienced. I called Jennifer, our angelic nurse practitioner, who prescribed Magic Mouthwash, an elixir to numb Paul's mouth. After fifteen minutes, it wore off and Paul chugged another mouthful. It would be another long day. To pass the time, we often walked. I come from a long line of walkers. The Fitzpatrick side of our family marched off everything from chicken pox to the common cold. My dad's solution to everything was either a dip in the ocean or a brisk hike.

> *To buoy Paul's mood and my own, we got out of the house today and head to the open fields of the Brooklyn Botanical Gardens. We sat under a grove of cherry trees and planned out the healing garden we wanted to plant some day. Paul smoked a bit of pot to stem the nausea. It helped for a while. He's so finicky about food smells and choices now. Later, at home, I cooked a comfort meal which seemed to do the trick—skinned chicken thighs marinated in onions, peas, and carrots with acorn squash baked in honey. He's sleeping now. Made it through another day.*
> —*October 2000*

One of the hardest things for me was watching Paul deal with some of the same symptoms I'd experienced—and being powerless to stop them. During his first chemotherapy session, I turned seasick and dizzy as I sat next to him. Nurse Ratchet injected Paul with the "red warrior,"

Adriomyacin. I didn't know whether it was sympathy pains or sense memory, but I felt my veins bubble.

> *I'm hanging by a thin thread today. I tried not to boss the nurses around at Paul's chemo visit. But I couldn't help asking (demanding?) "Popsicles, when should he get the fucking Popsicles?" I felt everyone stare as my voice echoed down the hall. Cold was known to be a protector against mouth sores during an infusion of this kind. I remember eating frozen fruit pops by the freezer-full during my treatments. As a been-there-done-that expert, I couldn't help but oversee the actions of the nurses. When Alicia, a kind nurse, described what Paul could expect over the next twenty-four hours, I barked, "I know what he's going to be feeling!"*
>
> —*October 2000*

"Laura," Paul told me the next morning, "I'm the patient now, not you. This is happening to *me*."

"I know, Paul," I cried, my jaw and shoulders tensed, "but it feels like it's happening to me too."

We were at a crossroads. As Paul got sicker, he withdrew from me and didn't even want to be touched. This deepened my own isolation. Touch comforted me, but it wasn't Paul's way to deal with illness. My head understood, but my heart was broken. I was devastated by his pulling away from me as we sat on the couch. *It's another loss they don't tell you about,* I thought to myself.

Thankfully, we were not alone. My mom came to all of Paul's treatments. She was never empty-handed and brought gift bags for each of us: a soft, downy neck pillow and thick, navy-blue socks for Paul and often, a piece of sparkly jewelry and flowers for me.

There were other signs of hope that I clung to. One day, Paul and I were ushered into another clinic room for a blood test prior to a treatment. A kind, familiar face greeted us. "Maria!" I shouted.

"What are *you* doing here?" she asked me. Maria had been my chemotherapy nurse not so long ago. I never expected to see her again, let alone in the position of caregiver for my husband. She told us she'd recently changed hospitals and had only been at Cornell for two weeks. I breathed a sigh of relief. In the middle of this teeming city was a Florence Nightingale I knew and trusted.

"Take care of him," I whispered before I left the room. Within seconds, my chemo unit despair had been lifted by an unexpected gratitude.

Going to work helped me through this period as well. I was on automatic pilot waiting for Paul's discomfort to pass. One morning, I got a call at the clinic just before a staff meeting. Unnerved, Paul was laughing and crying so hard he could hardly get the words out. "I'm balding all over," he sputtered, "even my butt hairs are falling out!" We agreed it was time for the head shave.

That Saturday, I dropped him off at the barbershop and circled the block. When he exited, his pale oval head looked so bare and unprotected in the afternoon sun. My heart stopped. He'd shaved his beard for me when I was undergoing chemo. But now, seeing his shorn scalp, I burst into tears. *He looks so different*, I wrote later, *only the eyes are Paul's*. As a wife and caregiver, this was the hardest thing I'd ever witnessed. I don't know how my parents and Paul did it when it had been my turn. In hindsight, I recognized that they too were in the throes of panicky love—waiting, watching, and worrying. Within days, Paul lost the rest of his body hair and with it, even more of his energy.

Underground Losses

"I feel like a frail old guy," Paul said one afternoon on the way to the hospital. We waited in traffic behind a long line of red lights on the FDR. "I have no strength," he continued, laying his head back. Since I'd known Paul, he'd always had great vigor and physical prowess. As a rock climber and a builder of houses, being a cancer patient with weakened veins and no hair *anywhere* really knocked him down. I could see it—and it hurt to watch. Losing my hair during chemo was a bizarre happening for me, but for Paul, it was akin to losing his maleness. Being zapped thirty-five times by radiation beams below the belt didn't help either.

Our physical relationship kept changing with these events too. The honeymoon was over. As a patient, Paul withdrew into himself to lick his wounds. I was the opposite. I sought affection when I didn't feel well. Even in between my own chemo appointments, I desired physical intimacy. On Paul's non-chemo days, I'd try to draw him out by lighting candles and putting on music. Paul often pulled away from me as though a chilly breeze had blown into the room. I knew with my head that Paul's body had changed because of the treatment. "Not my heart," he tried to reassure me. Fatigue drained him of energy *and* libido. After being rebuffed again, I'd slip out of bed and cry in our narrow city bathroom not wanting him to know how deeply I hurt. I poured out my fears into my notebook: *Will we ever be like we used to be? Will Paul ever find me attractive and sexy again?*

Now, years later, I can look back on that time with the healing balm of distance. Our bodies and psyches were permanently altered by the cancer and the side effects of treatment. That was real. Both of us kept wanting to go back to the days when we were carefree lovers dancing in the garage before our wedding. I missed the way we were and secretly felt robbed of a longer honeymoon period. Conversations about this were painful and awkward and often ended in tears streaming down our faces. "I'm in survival mode, Laura," Paul told me. "Give me time."

This was a place of hidden, subterranean losses. The aftershocks of treatment rumbled unspoken through our daily routine. This, we each carried in our hearts alone. Recovering a sex life was a taboo subject, even in the support group I joined. You could hear a pin drop when I broached the subject one day. My friends couldn't relate either. If they weren't having sex, it was because of kid exhaustion or heavy workloads. Four months passed—then six. Flipping through *Cosmopolitan* magazine while I was having my hair trimmed didn't help. "Most American couples reported having sex two–three times a week," read the glossy headline. My stomach lurched. Did that include cancer couples too? There was no easy-to-read map in this wounded place. I feared we were lost, but I hung on to what I knew about love. We'd already come so far.

> *Love right now is about finding intimacy in the small things: holding hands across the café table at Sotto Voce, Paul's palm pressing gently on the small of my back as we entered the room, walking along Seventh Avenue arm in arm, sharing a tender kiss goodnight. Patience is my guide.*
> —December 2000

As the willow leaves turned from green to gold outside our kitchen window, I crossed off the days on our calendar. This was a hope-filled act. As we approached the end of his treatment, Paul had more body scans. Finally, after biting my nails down to the quick again, Paul was told he was *clean*. I felt hope for the very first time since all this had started months ago. "It's as good as it gets; this is *curable*," commented Paul's teenage oncologist. I posted his words on our refrigerator.

Unwanted Commitments

Paul's healthy report took a while to sink in. Our emotional rollercoaster continued. I wasn't prepared to hear the clinical words like *follow-up* and *surveillance* for a second time. It never occurred to me that Paul, like me, would need to be *under surveillance* too. There were *still* no guarantees for either of us. As cancer survivors, each of us faced the uncertainty of tomorrow more directly than most.

"How often are my checkups?" Paul asked as I took notes.
"Every three months for two years," Dr. Mary told us.
"What about children?"
"Wait two years at least," she recommended.

> *This last bit of news swept over me like a tidal wave. What a commitment this damn follow-up schedule is. More and more doctors, waiting rooms, appointments, anxiety, body checks. And on top of it all, we got the take-home message to keep our hopes of a family under wraps. Paul and I assumed we'd have kids after this. I pictured myself at dawn in a rocking chair holding a baby with curly brown hair like my own. Paul told me he wanted a child to play baseball with in the yard. One step at a time says Mom. I'm jumping ahead too fast.*
> —January 2000

The picture of our new reality as cancer survivors, however, changed these daydreams. Grief surged in shifting currents of undertow. Years later, I've learned to accept that the commitment we made to each other was to much more than the drudgery of hospital appointments.

In a deeper sense, it was a long-term commitment to healing, to making choices that fed our bodies and nourished our souls. That is the world we live in, side by side. And it didn't have to include children to make us a family. We'd have enough to handle between the two of us, but back then, I wasn't ready to admit all of this to myself.

House Hunting

So, like newly released prisoners from Alcatraz, we planned our escape from New York City. With Paul's chemotherapy and radiation treatment behind us and mine a distant memory, we imagined our future full steam ahead. My hair and energy were back. Tight, curly ringlets fell around my ears. Paul's hair bristled with new salt-and-pepper growth. With life on the upswing, Paul even resumed taking art classes at the Art Students League in Manhattan. Of course, the deeper process of recovery and healing took many months and years to unfold, but the neon lights of trauma mode were behind us.

Little by little, we began to live—and dream again. We wondered daily about where we'd move to. *How do we want to live our lives now?* we asked ourselves. Paul and I talked into the night about that moment in time where we could take things for granted again. It's the place where normal people spend their lives. For the person with cancer, you can't imagine anything beyond the present moment. Now, with Paul's rounds of medical treatment over, we could pay attention to more ordinary concerns. Rather than scheduling the next radiation appointment, we worried about other real-life things like adding up our pennies for a down-payment, keeping up with the credit cards, and having friends over for a casual dinner. In between Paul's carpentry jobs around the city and my grading of student reports, we combed the Internet for a fixer-upper. We needed to find another place to call home.

> *It seems to be part of our healing to plan and imagine a different life for ourselves. We've been to the edge of doom and back. Each day feels like an*

> *extra gift. Now, house hunting, not chemo, is our new adventure.*
>
> *—February 2000*

We were elated at the prospect of moving to an affordable home somewhere in New England. My parents generously offered to help us with a down payment when we found what we wanted. Without them, we'd still be squatters in a Brooklyn apartment building.

While house hunting, I made the final decision to resign from Teachers College. It was a painful choice to make. I loved the university life, my colleagues and students, and the streets of the Upper West Side campus. But we sought a calmer, less hectic place to heal our lives and begin again. My career took a back seat. So I licked the envelope of my resignation letter and dropped it off at the department chair's office. Simultaneously, I mailed out résumés to schools in Massachusetts and Connecticut. I even went on a few interviews in both states just to keep my options open. Our new life lay somewhere beyond the Triborough Bridge.

I fell madly in love with most of the houses we saw—none of which were in our limited price range. Then, one blustery March day, we returned to take a second look at a collapsing bungalow we'd seen near beautiful Rogers Lake in Old Lyme, Connecticut. My folks lived twenty-five minutes down the road. We made an offer and signed the papers. For seventy-five thousand dollars and still remaining on a shoestring budget, we bought a half acre of overgrown, weedy countryside. Coming from a walk-up in Brooklyn, this modest ramshackle cottage was heaven. Paul had work to do!

> *Paul's in design mode with the renovation plans for the house. Today, he built a 3-D model out of foam core spending hours on roof lines, windows, and gardens for our new home. The dollhouse model sits on our coffee table wedged in between packing boxes, masking tape, and piles of papers. We'll even have a new zip code. Hope is in the air.*
>
> *—March 2000*

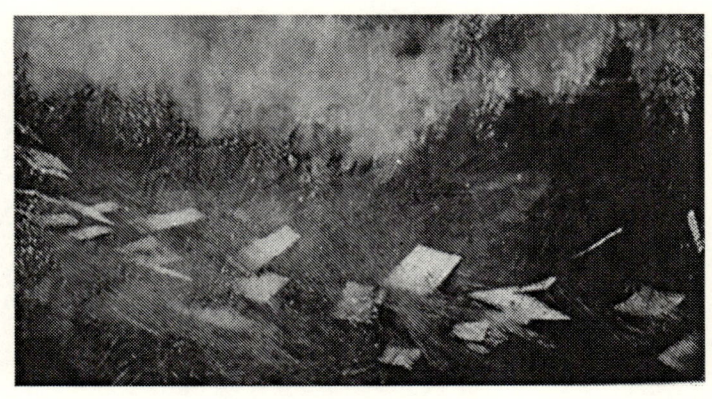

*Not knowing when the dawn will come
I open every door.*

—Emily Dickinson

Season 3

My Turn—Again

Round Three: Recurrence

Our excitement at moving to Connecticut was growing. We'd be closing on our house soon and saying good-bye to our work lives and friendships in New York. We now managed one another's medical checkups in between the packing of boxes. *Moving on* was our daily mantra. Cartons were piling up in the study in preparation for our upcoming move only weeks away. I even threw my wig into the trash bin on the sidewalk along with the other clutter we'd been collecting. Underneath all the frenetic energy was our unspoken desire to leave cancer far behind.

Nearly six months after Paul finished his last radiation appointment, I went for a midtown checkup to my oncologist. It was to be my final appointment before I transferred my medical care to Connecticut. Both of us had to find new physicians once the dust settled.

On this fateful day, we chatted with Dr. M. for a few moments about Paul's recent recovery and my own steady health. One minute we were on cloud nine at Dr. M.'s recommendation to us, and in the next, life changed on us again.

> *In slow motion, I see us smile in Dr M.'s wood-paneled office as she talked with us before examining me. She gave us the green light on having a baby! She even encouraged us with stories of other cancer patients who went on to have healthy children. One local physician she knew implanted an ovary in a woman's forearm and harvested some eggs. Paul said, "Wow, I think that's the best news I've ever heard!" We could hardly wait to leave the office for home so we could get cracking some eggs of our own.*
>
> *—June 2001*

With a quick kiss to Paul, I turned and followed Dr. M. into her tiny examining room. "I'll be out in a minute," I said. Seconds later, I sat on her steel table shivering in a cotton gown, her physician fingers touching a swollen lump in my neck the size of a horsefly bite. *Ouch*, I winced. I thought it was just a pimple when I noticed it in the shower the day before. I watched Dr. M.'s face harden into a cool, clinical mask. Her chatty warmth evaporated along with her smile as she told me to see a specialist for further testing. By that time, Paul was flipping pages in the waiting room. He stood up as he saw my petrified face. What began as an innocuous doctor's visit turned into another cancer diagnosis for me—this time, *recurrence*, a word I'd never even heard of before.

"I'm so sorry, Laura," Paul whispered into my ear as we walked hand in hand into the crowds along Seventy-second Street. I squeezed his fingers as a cold sweat formed on my brow. In spite of having lost my breast, enduring chemo drugs coursing through my body for months, being faithful to checkups, and nursing an ailing husband, the corrupt cells traveled into my neck and chest anyway, like poison ivy popping up in a tended garden. It was hard to put a stiff upper lip on this one. There simply were no guarantees.

> *Déjà vu. I'm reminded of the waiting game—that limbo place where your mind takes over and you don't know how much to be concerned, if at all, or whether you're being paranoid. We won't know the final test results for a few days. Shit. What if it is a recurrence? I'm going to stamp that word out of my mind until we hear for sure. Paul's good at that. Packing up will be therapeutic. We're moving anyway, whatever happens.*
>
> "We have to go on with our lives, Laura," Paul assured me.
>
> *—June 2001*

Within days, the results were in. The cancer was back in my chest and neck. There was no way to soften the blow. Replaying the week's news, I felt a cold sweat breaking out on my forehead again. Breast cancer was back for a third time—a *third* time. Only this time, they called it a *Recurrence* with a capital "R" for Raw Deal. Time stopped as we reconsidered our options. I feared what the news would do to my folks.

Cards poured into our mailbox, reminding me we weren't alone. Some friends knew just what to say. I had no words left.

Dear Laura and Paul,
 I wish this whole thing were behind you although not as much as you wish it I'm sure. But I wanted to remind you that this isn't payback for being ungrateful about anything, this is not the dark cloud that must come with all sunshine—it just is. No fault, no blame, no cosmic meaning. I promise. You can get through this and be happy.
Love always,
Cath

Dear Laura and Paul,
 Once more I'm heading to Brooklyn filled with only hugs to give and fears to share. Remember that we are together on this journey, regardless. It is a blessing to be part of your lives. We're so happy you're moving to CT. I want to welcome you into our home for as long as you need it! I think we can be a refreshing stopover for you as you recover and rebuild your lives.
We love you,
Mom and Dad

Moving Day

So, in spite of my recurrence and unpredictable prognosis, we moved ahead with our house plans. Days passed in a flurry of fear and packing. I answered phone calls from our lawyer handling the closing just moments after being prepped for a bone scan to determine the extent of the cancer. I wrote in my journal what I couldn't say out loud:

> *I have a black cloud over my head. How did this happen after everything we've been through? I don't deserve this. Does recurrence mean I'm going to die?*
> *—July 2001*

Packing took our minds off my third diagnosis. Taped up and labeled for storage was my wedding china, gold-rimmed with tea roses; Paul's thirty-six-inch printing press ordered during his chemo treatment; boxes of books and bookshelves built by Paul for our library-closet; two couches; the maple table inherited from my grandmother; one computer; and a rustic coffee table. We made two piles for the movers: one for long-term storage and the other, clothes and possessions we needed in the short-term while living at my folks.

Moving day finally arrived. TV-sized boxes were stacked up on the sidewalk early that morning. Our gentle Mexican landlord helped us carry things out to the car for our final good-byes. With a spider plant wedged between our two front seats, I turned to catch a last quick glimpse of my Brooklyn neighborhood in the rearview mirror. In a few hours, the moving van would meet us in my parents' Connecticut driveway. I've never been back.

Letting my mind wander, I counted up the fifteen years that I'd lived in New York City. Home was Manhattan for many years before

I moved out to cheaper digs in Brooklyn. All told, I spent my twenties and half of my thirties in New York. It's where I learned to grow up. After graduating from college in Boston, I left for the Big Apple, clueless as to what I wanted to do with my life—or who I was meant to be. I dabbled in a social work degree, tried the family car business, and finally settled into a career in education, dialing 1-800-TeachNY one cold February day. I finished a master's degree at New York University. My new career as a speech-language pathologist led me to schools in East Harlem, Greenwich Village, and then, finally, uptown to Morningside Heights and Teachers College at Columbia University.

I was proud of who I'd become, and I loved the wildness of New York, the faces from around the world that I saw every day as I jogged the three-mile loop around Prospect Park. I loved my bagel store, the corner butcher who sold the biggest meatballs, and standing in the rain on Saturday mornings waiting for half-price tickets to a Broadway musical. On my way to the subway each morning, I smelled the honey raisin buns from our Windsor Terrace bakery. New York is where I grew up. It's there I lost friends (and myself) only to find truer ones. It's where I learned to say no to people who dragged me down and said yes to the love of my life.

But now, sitting in bumper-to-bumper traffic, I was more than ready to say my farewells to the Big Apple—to my job, to my friends and cousins, to the hospitals we'd grown to know too well. I hoped there was less cancer in Connecticut. While Paul drove northbound along the New England Thruway and talked of house designs, I double-checked our plans. The pulse of the car motor softened my anxiety as my dashboard list of to-do's grew as long as the road ahead. I turned another page in my journal and scribbled:

> *1. Me:*
> *Unpack some boxes and find toothpaste.*
> *Meet Monday morning with my new medical team and start radiation at St. Raphael's Hospital in New Haven.*
> *Pick up prescription for Zanax.*
> *Breathe. Try not to think too much.*

2. Paul:
Work on the house full-time as architect and builder.
  Keep sense of humor while managing life with in-laws.
  Breathe.
3. Boxes:
Put in storage and forget about them (for years).
4. Health Insurance:
Remember to pay nine hundred dollars a month under COBRA plan until new job starts in September. Live off of organic macaroni and cheese and my parents.
                              —July 2001

The gravel in my parents' driveway crunched loudly as we pulled in. My folks hugged us and helped unpack our things in their first-floor bedroom, our temporary home. With their help, we tackled just about everything on my list. I started radiation treatment within days of our arrival. There was no time to waste.

The Miracle Jar

My days were occupied with daily hospital visits and keeping my fears at bay. An X-ray revealed not only a fractured clavicle, but cancer in the bone. Another shock coursed through me. I swallowed another Zanax. The gravity of my recurrent disease settled in, an unbidden nightmare. "We have lots of things we can do," said Dr. B., my new oncologist, "but there is no cure." Up until this moment, I had assumed that a cure was possible.

> *I walked up close to the screen and stared at the white, cloudy markings on the black-and-white film. Then I saw Paul's face turn chalky white. Falling on the heels of Paul's recovery from lymphoma, we're desperate for hope—for a miracle. Peach fuzz had just grown in on Paul's head! Now it was my turn to be sick—again. Am I going to make it this time?*
> —July 2001

I remember when my sister phoned and in tears asked, "How can your body take any more of this?"

"It will. I'm strong," I replied.

But was I? I reviewed my life. It seemed upside down. I'd resigned from my big-time university job to move to the woods of Connecticut. There I was, tied up in knots, surrounded by boxes and cancer, and terrified of what the next day's MRI would show.

The course of my initial radiation sessions for this third bout with cancer paralleled the journey of Lance Armstrong's trip up mountains on his bike. I hungrily followed the news of Lance's yellow-shirted ride to the finish line in the Tour de France. I cut out his picture from the *New Haven Register* and placed it in my leather wallet like a teen-age fan. The look on his face often brought me to tears. It was brave and rugged and victorious. I prayed it was how I would look when my cancer was gone.

> *I passed a billboard along the highway to St. R.'s today. A woman about my age was smiling. In the foreground was written the headline: "Diagnosis: Breast cancer. Prognosis: Grandmother." Will that ever be me?*
> —*August 2001*

Radiation treatment was easier physically than the relentless regimen of chemotherapy, but the daily grind of back-and-forth visits to the hospital was rigorous, and a deep fatigue set in. Paul told me to remember that our love grounded us—despite the shifting earth beneath our feet. "Soon enough, it will be behind us," he said. "Soon enough."

> *My life has changed so much I didn't know where I was when I woke up in the morning or what has happened to my body. Our life seemed like a speeding car careening out beyond our control. We've just been to another doctor's office, a pulmonologist for my shortness of breath.*
> —*September 2001*

I stopped writing. There was too much going on in my days to relive it on the page at night. The most I could manage was a few scribbles on scrap paper stuffed into a Miracle Jar, a recent gift from my mom. Sitting on my parents' porch overlooking the marsh, I'd write out my fears and stuff them in the jar. This new practice was a life-saving one. Was it possible to ask for too many miracles? I ran my finger along the word *Miracles* on the front of the jar. The jar was a solid container of swirling waves of blue, its dappled clay ridges cool to my touch. I imagined it was deep enough to hold not only my worries but my dreams as well. Hastily, I'd jot down requests on bits of paper.

For a CURE.
Remission for us BOTH, forever.
To grow old with Paul.
To finish radiation and get well again.
To be cancer free—after my bone scan today.
Paul's PET scan was clear. <u>Great</u> news!

Another day, I wrote on index cards and added more practical concerns to the mounting pile inside the jar:

Hope my new job works out.
Money needed for Home Depot bills.

Most cards were written in my own chicken scratch, but then I noticed Paul and my mom slipped in petitions of their own. I pulled out a few to sneak a peek one day. "There are no rules," I'd told them. "Anything goes. Write whatever's on your heart." In bold, block lettering, I recognized Paul's artistic hand.

MANY ANNIVERSARIES AND HEALTH FOR US BOTH. PLEASE.

Mom, in her neat, gentle cursive, wrote:

For Laura's clean tests today.

It hurt to see their handwriting. Their wishes were simple—like mine. While living with my folks for those months, my mom taught me a thing or two about miracles. "Miracles are everywhere," she told me on one of our morning walks. "I think they're like dreams," she said. "It's a miracle you moved here to be near us, that we could be a part of your getting well."

As the summer passed along in doctor's appointments, I kept up with the Miracle Jar, using it as a journal. I wrote more legibly as the weeks passed by. My neck spots shrank under the gaze of the radiation beams, and my grip on my own illness relaxed. My body was responding to treatment! I began to pen prayers for other family members and friends. My world opened and light poured in.

> *For my cousin Larissa and her medical tests.*
> *For Stephanie, Tom, and their newborn baby boy.*
> *For David.*

It felt good to worry about other people for a change. Up until now, I could only worry about myself or Paul.

My radiation days had a rhythm, centered on my Miracle Jar and the lively hospital waiting room. It was all I could handle. I had no idea how I'd add work to my list when the school year started after Labor Day. One patient was always beginning treatment, while another one celebrated her completion. Graduates often left trays of homemade brownies or oatmeal cookies for the rest of us. Some left cards with thoughtful inscriptions like, *If I can make it, so can you* or *Thanks for being there for me.* These notes reminded me of my secret jar musings.

> *Strange how talking to fellow patients about the weather, exchanging skin cream tips, or quietly turning the pages of a well-worn* People *magazine makes me almost feel I'm at the corner hair salon. This waiting room is part support group, part coffee clutch. It's a hangout, the one place where I feel I belong.*
> —August 2001

It was at the hospital that I met Sally—a grandmotherly volunteer with a bright smile. Sally was in remission from bone cancer. "A miracle!" she told me, her eyes shining.

Yes, it is *a miracle,* I thought.

"Even though cancer went to your bones, it will be gone one day—like mine is," Sally whispered. From my research, I knew that I was in a dangerous place as far as cancer staging went. No one said the words *stage four* to me, but that is what cancer is called when it enters the bone. I was terrified of what that meant and spoke of it to no one but my counselor—and now, Sally. She was someone else whose cancer had spread into the bones. That night, I scribbled to the Miracle Jar: *Let my bones heal like Sally's.* She'd given me hope like no one else had.

It dawned on me that I hadn't given much thought to whom I was miracle-sending. I wasn't sure if I wrote to the Universe, to God, or to Life, but the act of writing my thoughts and dropping them into the jar felt true—holy, like praying, like relief. I heard a line from Isaiah in my pleadings: *breathe life into these dry bones.* And when my breath would turn shallow in the night, I'd remember again, *breathe life into these dry bones—and Sally's.*

Morning Poem

Diving in for an early swim,
I taste the cold, salty waves of September's ocean.
I dress,
racing to my car with Earl Gray in my cup,
minutes to spare to get to work.
I'm scared.
Of losing this life.
Of missing our dance in the garage
at dawn,
Of holding your whiskered face
under moon rivers.
When you have so much to live for,
death comes hard.
I'm running out of time,
forgetting to enjoy this moment,
the lightness of rustling wind through bamboo.
The opposite of terror
is fearlessness.
Or maybe it's all within us.
This beauty, this fear, this being human.

Where the Wild Things Are

I was more than halfway through my radiation treatment with only two weeks left to go. Since early September, I'd been working at a local elementary school. My daily regimen included leaving school after lunch each day for my afternoon appointment at the hospital. The pressure of managing my new job as a school speech-language pathologist and moonlighting as a radiation patient was exhausting. But we needed the income *and* the health insurance. While I was at work, Paul poured a new foundation for our house. We continued to live at my parents'.

At work, I did my best to meet the demands of seeing forty kids for therapy each week and managing piles of paperwork. I didn't have my own office space anymore—just a cramped corner in a dusty alcove of the special ed room. The memory of my spacious, book-lined office at Teachers College was a hidden thorn of loss in my side. However, I was grateful for this new school administration. They did their best to accommodate my precarious health needs so I persevered. I fell into bed like a zombie each night.

On Tuesday, September 11, my shaky resolve cracked. I trembled uncontrollably as I drove toward the oncology ward at St. Raphael's Hospital. Gripping the black leather steering wheel, I clung to bits of news on the radio about the horror unfolding: planes crashing, Tower One collapsing, smoke billowing. I dialed the hospital from my cell phone. In between the sounds of sirens, screams, and talk of *the missing* on National Public Radio, I waited for someone to pick up the phone. What a bizarre backdrop to my own inner chaos, my own war with the terrorist cancer cells attacking my body. I was surprised when a nurse answered my call.

"Should I still come in today?" I asked her.

"Of course," she replied. "See you when you get here."

Phew, the oncology unit was status quo even though much of the world had come to a startled stop. My cancer was still a priority regardless of the day's events. Despite the fact it was a *cancer* routine, there was something oddly reassuring about it on a day like this one—structure amidst the chaos.

I regretted my bravado on the phone with Paul. He'd offered to come with me today. But I wanted to spare him more grief and suggested he stay at work. Even though I could have used the extra support, it was hard for me to ask for what I needed when everyone was already so considerate of me. Often, Paul and I protected each other from the undertow of fear lurking under our daily routines. I recalled how I'd held Paul the night before and listened to his sobs. He clung to me, tears running down his cheeks. It was the first time since my re-diagnosis that Paul gave voice to his fears: "I'm afraid to lose you. Please don't die," he whispered.

Once I'd entered the hospital, I found consolation in the familiar rhythm: changing into a worn gray hospital gown, glancing in the dressing room mirror, finding an empty chair, and flipping through magazines. On this day, I sat down next to Beverly, a fellow patient I'd seen the day before. We'd each heard the news and shared our New York stories while we waited. She'd lived there once too. We agreed that the freakish events at Ground Zero mirrored the out-of-control feeling we were living with in our own lives.

Our talk was interrupted by a kind voice over the loudspeaker. "Laura, c'mon back."

I met Teresa and Susan, my technician friends, in the radiation chamber with a friendly hug. We usually exchanged "how are you's" and other pleasantries as I climbed onto the narrow steel table. They configured the machines to zap me at just the right angles and then covered me with a warm blanket. Tiny blue tattoos graced my neck and chest for this purpose. But today, our talk was of the Towers. None of us could imagine that the smoky devastation on TV was real.

I shivered and closed my eyes to relax during my treatment. I'd been taught to do visualizations and breathed in deeply, counting to five. *One, two, three, four...* Today, it was harder than usual to shut the door on my mind's chatter. Feeling my lungs expand, I tried to picture myself on a Cape Cod beach bathed in brilliant sunlight as rays of gold and pink zapped the cancer cells away. No luck. Instead, I stared at the ceiling and trembled in the shadowed light. For a few moments, I longed to forget it all—the cancer, September 11, everything ...

Daydreaming, I found myself sitting on a wooden stool in our blue and yellow Brooklyn kitchen. In calmer days, Paul and I often climbed up the rickety steps to our *tar beach* roof and gazed at the distant view of lower Manhattan. The Twin Towers stood majestically in the distance. I couldn't imagine a hole in the ground where once such life stood. My heart pounded with my memories. The voice of a nurse broke through my reverie. *Time to go*. Climbing off the radiation table, I waved my good-byes and retraced my steps to the waiting room. I massaged a soothing ointment into my radiated skin and dressed quickly.

Pushing the hospital door open, I was surprised that the sun was out. Tilting my face to the sky, I gulped fresh air like it was water and walked to my car. At that moment, the fatigue and shock of the day hit me—this one day. Turning on my car engine, I heard a journalist's weary voice give an update on conditions in Manhattan. I reached to crank the radio louder and stopped. I couldn't take any more news of the world's madness. All I wanted was the quiet safety of my own car—and to get home to my family waiting around the dinner table for me.

* * *

Days passed. While the wider world recovered slowly from the chaos at Ground Zero, we watched the cancer cells in the lymph nodes of my neck and chest disappear. My collarbone, too, had responded to the intensity of my treatment. Over the six-week course of radiation, I'd been zapped a total of thirty-five times. And then, it happened—a real miracle. Somehow, under the strong rays of radiation and drugs to keep my ovaries quiet, my cancer disappeared. "No evidence of disease" was stamped in black ink on the pathology report. With a pink magic marker, I jotted down my medical headlines and opened the Miracle Jar:

I give thanks for so much: today's hopeful news! For tonight's party, my family, and the end of my radiation!!!!

Recovery Notes

During the two years post-recurrence, I crossed the threshold of a new phase of treatment. I continued to have monthly visits to my oncologist for an infusion of medication to keep my bones strong and prevent recurrence. Those oncology checkups and periodic scans were only part of my wellness steps at the time. From a counselor at the hospital, I received one-on-one support. From her, I learned to deal with the residue of trauma that remained in my heart. And to make better choices.

Fortunately, I had many resources offered to me through the Integrative Medicine Department at St. Raphael's. I'd checked out several support groups in the area and liked the one offered at the hospital called the Life Enhancement Group. This circle of support was for cancer survivors in all stages of cancer diagnosis and recovery. Each session began with a meditation, one of many life-enhancers I learned to integrate into my life.

> *I'm feeling better each day. My radiation pneumonia is gone along with that damn cough. Heading into my group this afternoon. Paul's meeting again with a group of guys to talk, too. We each need support now beyond what we can give each other. And the free parking is a rare cancer perk.*
> —November 2001

True healing would take much longer than I'd expected. For one thing, I was physically and emotionally depleted. I was unable to resume full-time work. With reluctance, I took a leave of absence from my new job and packed up my school office again. Healing was my priority. It had to be.

> *A new member to the group today asked me what stage my cancer was. Without missing a beat, I said, "I'm in the healing stage; that's where I am." I'm not here to compare tumor notes, I thought, but to figure out how to cope and move on with my life!*
> —*February 2002*

Through group and individual support, I began to see a future again with Paul beyond my present health concerns, but fallout from cancer still rippled into our days.

"I wished things were different than they were," I'd admitted at a subsequent group meeting. Unexpectedly, things would come crashing through; I'd be overcome by grief at a baby shower or grow anxious upon hearing of another friend's recurrent cancer. It didn't help that we were rejected as prospective parents one Monday night by a local adoption agency. We'd blown our chances right out of the water when the presenters heard about our health histories.

> *I'm struggling with accepting the Plan B of our lives. I keep looking back. Seeing those families with their adopted toddlers the other night, I'm wanting what I can't have. We decided to say good-bye to the sperm bank, too. It's not going to happen. Paul said all he cares about is our being together. I soaked his shirt with my sobs. I've had to say good-bye to so much. We both have. Bottom line: I don't want to be a cancer patient anymore.*
> —*November 2002*

These decisions didn't happen overnight. It helped to move into our own house. Moving out of my folks' and into our own digs signaled another new phase of healing: Moving on. Instead of talking about cancer, we talked about light fixtures. Instead of waiting for test results, we bought sinks for both bathrooms. We picked out clay tile for the front and back hall. Paul built bookshelves, and I emptied out more boxes. I bought violets and ivy to fill our new bay window.

This house mirrors us in many ways with its unfinished walls and our unfinished stories, I thought. Paul worked tirelessly to make our little shingled house a home. He worked so hard he needed shoulder surgery two days after we moved in. "I've carried every nail and every stick of lumber in here from Home Depot *myself!*" Paul announced. Life was not dull.

> *An anniversary day to celebrate! Two years ago today was my recurrence. It seems light years ago now. We spent a lazy day at home. Paul made a fire to take the chill out of the air. We drove to our favorite ice cream shop and later, walked along the beach. So much to be grateful for ...*
> *—June 2003*

With time, I began to trust my body again. I had renewed energy to focus on my career too. I joined a school system and a private practice near our home. I was trying to befriend my life, as author Naomi Rachel Remen wrote in *Kitchen Table Wisdom*, and not always be on the defensive against cancer. I also traveled to New Mexico to write and discovered a group of kindred spirits there.

> *Where do I find hope these days?*
> *In the words "rock solid" from my doctor.*
> *In the message of another friend's remission.*
> *In the meows of our adopted kitten, Daisy.*
> *In working with kids.*
> *With my new writing friends.*
> *I'm beginning to trust that I am beating this thing. My body is well.*
> *—August 2003*

A Letter to My Doctor

November 2003

Dear Dr. B.,

    Waiting for my oncology appointment today, I thought about what it's been like being your patient over these years. And I share in the sadness you must be feeling over your wife's failing health from breast cancer. With you as my oncologist, I've felt a sense of safety, compassion, and interest from you. You've always given me your full attention and expertise. You've even followed the progress of my house and laughed with me when I complained that it was taking too long.
    By now, I'm sure I'd know your footsteps anywhere—the determined shuffle and fast-paced tap, tap, and tap of your heels touching the speckled linoleum at lightning speed. "How much longer will I have to keep coming here?" I'd asked you during those initial visits after my recurrence.
    "Forever," you said in a matter-of-fact tone. Your choice of wording reverberated like an echo for many days afterward. I didn't want an oncologist to be a steady presence in my life. I still don't. A dentist is one thing, but a cancer doctor quite another!
    The squeak of your black leather soles and creak of a neighboring door always signals your arrival. Your feet pause reflectively across the hall to record a patient's prognosis into your hand-held cassette. "Hello," you said to me in a booming baritone. "How are you doing today?" The door closed behind you with a confidential click. You sat on a shiny round chair with wheels, your toes touching the tiled floor.
    "So, how's everything going? What's new?" you asked, head lifting to meet my eyes. Papers rustled again as you flicked through my thick

chart. Any wayward symptom or distress or bone ache and you'd ask more questions, examine me, and order more tests. No time is wasted under your watchful gaze. You've kept on top of things.

"Everything's great. I feel great," I said. It was true except for the boulder in my stomach. *Thud.* We are both in a battle with cancer. I am winning mine right now, but you are losing your wife, Barbara, to this same disease. The latest news I heard through the grapevine—she's back in the hospital again. My blood pressure leapt a notch or two as I prepared myself for our recent appointment. I even rehearsed what I'd say. I worried about whether I'd see you at all in case you needed to be by your wife's side instead of at the office. Her cancer has steadily gained ground.

Today, I finally asked you, "How are *you* doing?" At my side was a gift bag containing a silky lemon-colored scarf for Barbara. I imagined she might be able to wrap it around her head and be soothed by its sun-drenched colors. Not wanting to be empty-handed when I saw you, it caught my eye as I stepped into the hospital gift shop. My mother taught me to always bring something in times of distress. This seemed like one of those times. I hoped to comfort you, and yet, I needed reassurance—for myself, too.

"My wife and I have known each other for over fifty years," you told me at a prior appointment, and "we even played together as children." Your voice wavered with pride, amazement, and something gravelly, shaken by grief. You shared how you'd dealt with the unknown timeline of her illness. "I've sought out short-term pleasures, planned trips we could look forward to. We've gone to the opera and renewed our subscription series. We never thought she'd make two more years, but she did!" you said standing up to leave.

On this morning, our visit was short. I'm doing well so there was no reason for a lengthy checkup. "I'm scared, for myself," I blurted out too loudly just as your hand reached for the doorknob.

Your weary eyes looked directly into mine. "I know." You nodded, sitting down again, feet planted heavily on the floor. "You have to remember that everyone's cancer is different. No two diseases are the same. You're doing well. Barbara's had this for many years."

I need to be reminded again and again of this truth. Every person's illness, like her life, is unique. Barbara's shoes are not mine. And yet she and I have walked similar paths—even met a few times in these clinic hallways. "Here," I stood nervously, handing you the present. "Please tell Barbara I've been thinking about her." I wanted to give you a hug but my feet were frozen. Your retreating footsteps filled the busy corridor.

I know that you can't predict the future, or even cure me. I also know that you've taught me how to live, despite the uncertainty of tomorrow. There are many things not in my control, or in yours, like your wife's disease or mine. But I've relied on the comfort that your skillful presence has offered, the quick clatter of your steps rushing up and down the unit. I appreciate deeply the thoughtful way you've explained the difference between me and other patients, the time you've taken to listen, part father figure, part physician.

Through your own wife's struggle, I've been afraid that you'd lose hope for me. I'll admit to even losing some hope in you. I'm reminded on this day that you, too, are only human. That's the secret. The hope I've searched for turns out to be different than the one I'd expected. My life isn't in your hands. As my doctor, you don't have all the answers—even though I walk through the door at every appointment still wishing for that 100% Duracell guarantee on long life. You do know that loving and living each day—with care—is the answer, no matter what happens tomorrow.

Thank you for everything.

With gratitude,
Laura

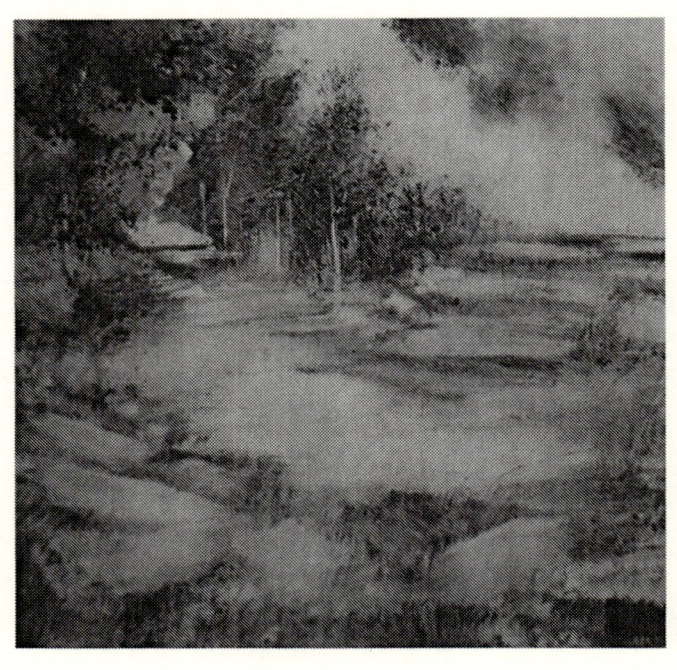

I dwell in possibility.
——Emily Dickinson

Season 4

Homecoming

This season is one of abundance. We're settling in to our lives and putting down roots. Both of us are in remission and comfortable there. The rhythm of work, family, and health is a balancing act. I know it is for everyone. Time is more fluid; reflections flow. A garden grows.

A Poem from Paul

I'm looking at you ...
When I open my eyes each morning,
When I fall from grace,
When I shine, when I falter ...
There is less to consider, more to gain
when I'm looking at you.
It's no small wonder that I've lasted this long.
No small wonder that we found each other.
The snow, the trees in winter,
the time it takes to go from there to here ...
I've been to places up high and climbed out over my world,
But when I look at you, I see the future ...
I see heart and love and joy and cinnamon buns by the fire.
Looking is cooking but seeing is freeing ...
Architecture, structure, dreams, schemes ...
Now and then,
then and when,
a question of time, a wish for sublime
my pun, the rhyme,
Is it full? Is it time?
To speak out, to speak up, to speak to ...
When I look out the window, Laura, I'm looking at us,
I'm looking at you.

All my love,
Paul

Ginkgo Day

Years ago, my mother gave me a favorite book of hers from her college days. *How to Know Trees* was required reading for her botany class. "Growing up as a city kid in Boston, all I knew was centered on the one elm tree that grew in our backyard," she told me. "If I was going to be a teacher, I thought I should know something about the woods."

Although out of date and worn, Mom's grassy-green book is among my treasures. As a former resident of Manhattan, I'd need all the help I could get in the garden. Paul is much more patient with pruning, planting, and potting than I am. Thoughts of landscaping used to be a far-off dream when cancer was in the foreground—not anymore. I open its yellowing pages for seeds of wisdom about the names of things growing in our small backyard. I read about oak and maple trees, ginkgo, and pines. *What new trees should we plant this season?* we wondered recently.

> *If I ignore the roof staging, abandoned tools, and ladders out back, our house looks almost finished these days with a heart wreath on our cherry-red front door. Sometimes I think I may never have a closet door or painted trim on my windows, but the garden is shaping up!*
>
> *—May 2004*

One of the things that caught our eye when we bought this property was the trees. Though the roof of this little house was collapsing, the trees formed a sheltering green canopy over us as we meandered through the yard. Walking here reminds me of when I was a child and my grandfather held my hand gently as we wandered through his New

England woods. We'd stop under a glowing beech, craning our necks to the sky through dark, velvet leaves. "You can read the health and name of a tree by its calling card, the leaf," he'd tell me.

Like a palm reader, I traced the lines in my own grown-up hand. *How much time do Paul and I have to enjoy our lives?* I wondered. Longevity, health, and gardening have been major themes in my marriage. I sift through them as I turn the rich soil for new trees and other plantings with a rusted garden hoe. Though our yard measures half an acre in between neighboring homes, it smells spacious with its fresh, mossy earth, over-ripened fruit trees, and an aging cedar.

Each spring, our ancient Chinese ginkgo tree begins to bud again. I can see its promising tips from the bay window in my kitchen. A small, carved birdhouse hangs from one of its branches—home to a family of robins each spring. The ginkgo, I learned in my mother's book, was considered a sacred tree of healing in Japan and often graced the monasteries of old. Ours stands thirty feet in height with outstretched, solid branches. Its half-moon-shaped leaves are like mini-parachutes that wiggle when the wind blows.

I remember one blustery morning in late autumn not so long ago. The world outside was deep crimson and burnished orange when a streak of yellow caught my eye from the upstairs bathroom window. We had only lived here for six months. "Paul, come quick! It's the ginkgo!" I yelled. A steady shower of saffron butterfly leaves fell from the tree.

"Listen," Paul said. "Can you hear that? It sounds like it's raining!"

A few moments later, with steaming mugs in our hands, we settled outside into blanketed beach chairs. The ginkgo's leaves continued to drop in front of us like a waterfall of golden feathers. Being in the moment was a gift I was often too busy to see, but not on this day. Within two hours, the rapid fire of falling leaves slowed to a trickle. Blue sky was visible through the branches—a moment of grace. Our first annual Ginkgo Day was born. I remember, too, when the flurry of leaves stopped.

> *Paul told me today that he was in the "fall" of his life. My heart sank. He's so depressed. More fallout? His dark mood reminds me there isn't a time line for*

> *healing. There are seasons of new growth, loss, and desolation for us, just like there are for our ginkgo.*
> —*October 2004*

At that time, we were in the throes of landscaping, but progress came to a standstill when Paul confided in me that he wasn't sure he could go to a nursery and buy saplings. "Do we have the time it takes to see them grow into real trees like other people?" Paul asked. His question hung in the air between us. "If I was younger, I'd plant seedlings and know my grandkids could climb their strong branches someday. But now? I'm fifty."

I knew Paul's fears. I shared them too. How much time did we have with each other in this life? Where were the guarantees we'd see any tree climb to the sky? "How much does it cost to buy fully grown ones? Let's at least go look, Paul. C'mon," I urged.

In the end, we compromised. One Sunday, when Paul's whistling returned, we visited a nursery a few miles from our house. We pushed metal carts up and down rows of pansies and impatiens. Annuals were my favorite. They offered immediate satisfaction to a weekend gardener like me.

The scent of morning dew and damp earth was in the air. We walked to the back of the grounds where the trees were in rows and eyed six-foot-tall cypress cedars, already on their way to new heights. "Look, Paul, these are *fast growers*," I said, reading the orange tag in my hand.

The owner, a mud-covered character in overalls, walked over to give us a hand.

"*Fast growers* mean you'll see healthy growth, maybe as much as twelve to twenty-four inches a year," he commented.

We bought as many *fast growers* as our pockets could handle. On a second cart, we placed two lilacs and a medium-sized flowering cherry tree, already blossoming pink. "We can enjoy their colors right now," I said.

More seasons have passed since that first Ginkgo Day. Back in our garden, crocus tips and the yellowing buds of forsythia bushes are welcoming signs of early spring. On the Internet, I read about temperature zones and years to maturity, about soil types and kinds of organic fertilizer. There are still days when the fear of losing what we have scares us to the point of paralysis. Some days, we can't quite hold our own after a routine CAT scan. Sometimes planting saplings and believing in the future is a gamble. Luckily, we take turns on this emotional seesaw and our periods of panic are fewer. Paul's arms around me bring me back into the moment, into what I *can* control, like which bulbs to plant and how to handle the over-friendly deer in our yard.

We're not alone in our struggle. One rainy, wet day, Dad offered to dig holes for the new trees we'd bought. "If I can't golf, I might as well get a workout," he said. My friend, Cathy, too, arrived from Boston to help replant flats of pansies into new window boxes.

In ten more years, God willing, our garden will burst with more branches of green to shelter us from the August sun and turn amber again with the frosty chills of October. A line from Rumi, the ancient thirteenth-century Sufi mystic and poet, comes to mind: "Be still, these trees are great prayers."

I pray Paul and I will share many seasons together, that our roots will grow deeper, that we will risk planting perennials next year, knowing that we may not see their rich blossoms as soon as we'd like, that time and nurturing and the weather will tell what happens in our garden, that we will risk loving each other even more with each passing season.

Piled up on our coffee table in the living room are our latest reads: a book Paul received from his sister, Ilene, on shade gardening; the latest issue of *Cottage Living* magazine; and my mom's college book, *How to Know Trees*. There is much more to learn.

I give thanks that today is a sure thing: watering our sweet peppers, weeding the dandelions, and making room for yet another evergreen tree.

Spa Secrets

I made a beeline for the spa. I was spending the weekend at a posh inn with other breast cancer survivors on a wellness retreat sponsored by our local hospital. Included in the price was a discount on spa services. The capital letters in the scented gold brochure really got me. I'm a sucker for gold. Paul dropped me off early so I'd have extra time to myself before the events of the weekend started. My heart pumped loudly in my chest as we pulled into the parking lot.

Head and shoulders, knees and toes, knees and toes ... I hummed the childhood tune to myself as I climbed the lobby steps. *Ahhh ...* After checking in and receiving my key, I stuffed my clothes and shoes in the locker and inhaled the aroma of rest—eucalyptus, lavender, and cinnamon. Slipping into cool turquoise flip-flops and a fluffy white terrycloth robe, I floated towards the Relaxation Room on a cloud. I poured myself a cup of lemon herbal tea and stretched out on a comfy wicker chaise. My eyes closed as I lay back on the downy pillow in the Relaxation Room, where with the other guests, I waited for my masseur to claim me. I wiggled my toes and purred contently like our yellow tiger cat in a sunspot.

At a $135.00 a pop for a facial, I didn't want to miss a second. My *provider*, as she was called by the front desk, entered a few minutes late and beckoned me to follow her. She seemed business-like but her smile was warm as I handed her my health questionnaire. While sipping my tea, I'd written the essentials on the nondescript form, putting a check mark next to the *cancer* word and *right mastectomy* under *surgical history*. I left out my tonsillectomy at age seven. It's always a toss-up for me how much to show and tell on these 1040-ish forms, but I figured since I only had my underpants on, my history would be somewhat obvious.

Provider Patricia took the clipboard from me without a glance as we entered the candlelit room and placed it on the counter before leaving again. I slipped under the downy sheets. *Maybe she'll read it later, I thought, while I'm dozing in a sweet lavender haze. Maybe she won't come in at all and I can just lay here for the weekend.*

A moment later, Patricia returned and silently worked on my face, shoulders, arms, and feet. She massaged and creamed my face and put gloves like oven mitts on my hands and toes. "Oooh, that feels great," I purred as she slipped my foot into another warm, soft mitten. Facials aren't just for faces anymore.

On my cheeks, nose, chin, and forehead, she rubbed layer after layer of creams and potions and a pumpkin mask that I'd agreed to pay extra bucks for. It was Halloween season after all, and my dry pores needed all the treats they could get.

As an herb-scented cloth was placed over my eyes and my cheeks were hardening with pumpkin du jour, Patricia's hands expertly worked their way down my neck onto my bony shoulders. This was the life. Her kneading fingers scouted out knots of tension and released them. She tapped a button on the floor with her shoe, and the lights went out. We were left in total darkness. I purred again. The warmth made me sleepy.

Suddenly, the lights clicked on in a flash of lightning as Patricia's hands touched my port, located under the skin above my left breast. "What's this?" she shrieked, her hands leaving my skin as though she'd touched dirty linen.

"Well," I struggled to find the words, "I've had breast cancer, and that's my port. It's for medication. But it's nothing to worry …"

She cut me off mid-sentence and blurted out harshly, "But I heard you shouldn't have a facial if you have cancer."

"Nnno, nnno," I stammered, "I'm not in active treatment now. I'm a ten-year survivor. Doing great. Don't worry."

I had a port surgically implanted under my skin after my recurrence. It was the size of a quarter and lay just below where my bra strap rested. I forgot it was even there. The port made getting shots and checkups easier since my veins no longer liked being poked and prodded—a remaining side effect of chemotherapy. I wanted it removed, but it was still useful for blood draws and medication. I hoped I wouldn't need it someday soon.

> *My face burned with more than pumpkin goo—with something like shame or anger, or both. I should have bolted out of there but wasn't thinking straight. Instead, I lay back down hoping to go back to images of me swimming in gentle turquoise waves.*
>
> *What a nightmare. My God, she was touching me like I was infectious.*
>
> *—October 2005*

Squish, I heard the rubbery sound of latex gloves. This was turning into a bad dream. Patricia's hands—now gloved—moved tentatively back to my shoulders then to more distant places like my arms and feet. The firmness of her touch faded into light, mechanical strokes. I felt fear in her clammy fingertips.

A few minutes later, Patricia announced the treatment was over and said she'd meet me outside. *Click.* The door closed. Sitting up, I blotted my eyes with a hand towel and quickly wrapped my robe around me. Some cream was left on one of my arms so I wiped that off too. With a nod to Patricia in the hall, I padded softly back to the locker room dizzy with embarrassment.

At dinner that night, I told my friends about what really happened during my expensive facial. Like the good friends that they were, they bolstered my spirits and helped me find the words:

"You go back there to that spa and speak to the manager."

"Get your money back!"

"Have that woman fired! I've never heard of such a horrible thing!"

"We'll go with you!"

In the end, I went by myself the next morning, my friends' voices in my heart. I got up my courage and pushed open the grand spa doors once again. The manager, a lovely, blonde thirty-something, ushered me into her small office. Behind her closed door, my humiliation and anger spilled out.

She listened with kind eyes and asked, "What can we do to make sure this never happens again?"

"Body image is a fragile thing," I said, "especially after the scars of cancer." Being treated with kid gloves (not rubber ones) is a must.

> *I left with a generous bag of apology filled with three hundred dollars worth of face creams, a cherry scented candle, and tea tree massage oil. I shared the contents of my bag with my retreat friends, and we covered our necks and faces with ginger gels and vitamin C eye serum. Apologies sometimes come in nice packages, huh?*
>
> *—October 2005*

Several days later, I received a salmon-pink note in the mail from the spa. In it was a gift certificate for the resort's signature caviar facial. The manager got the message. Provider Patricia, for all of her ignorance and lack of tact, reminded me how afraid we all are of death and illness. The myths and misconceptions about cancer can make us turn away from each other and run in the opposite direction, as if cancer were somehow transmittable through the air or by knowing someone too well.

Licking the envelope on a thank-you card, I thought of enclosing a note to Patricia too. It would read something like this: *Cancer isn't contagious, only fear is.* Life's lessons are funny this way. Who knew I'd go in for a facial and come out with a voice? And I swear my skin is smoother than it ever was.

An Anniversary Letter to Paul

Turning the pages of our wedding album, I see my favorite picture of us. We are sitting on a Cape Cod jetty in our wedding finery looking out at the horizon. I am sitting on your lap with my veil billowing behind us like a kite dancing on the wind. There is such promise in our proud, strong bodies. We'd been married for an hour. *Husband* and *wife* were two new words which sounded strange and wonderful in our mouths. Just a moment before, we'd stood under the *chuppah* you built for this day. My mom led us all in a joyous, sacred celebration. Remember how she beamed as she said those words we'd been waiting to hear, "You may now kiss each other as husband and wife"? We floated down the aisle to the sounds of violins, applause, and the ringing of bells. (Thanks to Kevin who snuck up to the belfry just in time.)

We'd already learned that life was shorter than we'd imagined. Our courtship days were a mad flurry of highs and lows. In this bridal photograph, we're braced for the unknown. My hair was still growing back in from the chemotherapy. Now it's long and wavy, down to my shoulders. Underneath the gorgeous gown of my dreams, I wore a strapless corset that held my newly reconstructed breast in place. You knew my scars and married me anyway. Facing the future from those rocky shores, we knew that we needed determination, effort, and the love of each other to build our new life, but neither of us expected it would be so hard.

The life lessons we've shared have brought us to the five-year hallmark. Today, our life has an easier rhythm. We're both living the three R's: remission, remission, remission. Can you believe our oncologists now share a practice together? Thankfully, our journey is one of wellness, not disease.

Recently, while you finished remodeling my parents' basement, I walked for miles on the beaches of my childhood: Corporation, Bay View, Chapin. Their names are like footprints in the sand for me. I am a child again writing letters at low tide with a stick and running into the lapping waves. It's summer vacation for me, and I am here at the Cape writing and walking to my heart's content. This is my summer of forty-two! Forty-two sounds adventurous, powerful, and celebratory—none of that over-the-hill baggage I struggled with at forty. Cancer has a way of jump starting crisis and makes you stare in the dark at yourself for longer than you think you can stand. But stand here I do, with pen in hand to chronicle our story and celebrate this moment in time.

Being here together, at the five-year marriage mark, I see the open road ahead of us. We've moved past the looking-back-wishing-it-were-different phase. Oh sure, there are still persistent, unanswered questions that we live with. But I've found that living with the questions is also about living with hope. The questions in my heart are open-ended ones now, and no answers will be found today:

Did we make the right choice to take care of ourselves rather than adopt children?

Will you make a career change and leave carpentry behind for your art?

Should I go back to graduate school or just keep writing?

Will we celebrate our twentieth wedding anniversary together?

These questions shape our days ahead as we heal forward. Thankfully, the fallout and aftershocks from cancer have receded. Your depression has lifted. I'm feeling less anxious about the unknown. We're lovers again, taking pleasure in our changed, mellowing bodies. You're dreaming of sailing a small wooden boat down the Connecticut River and out into the wide waters of Long Island Sound. I'm giving workshops on writing and healing. We're in a good place—a place of safety, partnership, and love, don't you think? A place wild and wonderful with, as Rilke says, the "winds of homecoming."

Happy Anniversary.

With big love,
Laura

My Ovary Party

When I stepped into Friends restaurant, I scanned the crowd for my sister, Julie. It took me a moment to realize the smiling faces of my family yelling "Surprise!" were for me. I knew my birthday had passed. *What's up?* I wondered. Small packages tied up in pink ribbons and balloons were on the table with the water glasses. I blinked back the tears. Paul pulled a chair out for me, and I sat down.

"Surprise!" my mother said as she handed me a shiny gift bag. "We wanted to lift your spirits." And with that introduction, my sister, Julie, recited her gift to me, a poem called, "A Night to Honor Your Insides."

I blushed. This was the eve of my oophorectomy. Although I'd grown accustomed to my dad and brothers saying the words *mastectomy*, *breast implant*, and *nipple*, talking about my ovaries was quite another matter. I was about to enter another operating room. This time, I would have my ovaries out. It was a precautionary move, a preemptive strike to clear out any risk factors *down there*.

Since my recurrent breast cancer was estrogen positive, removing any source of estrogen was the goal of my treatment. For years now, I'd had shots of Lupron, a drug used to keep my ovaries quiet. I knew the hot flashes, tissue dryness, and mood swings of menopause well, but this drug was relatively new with little data on long-term side effects. Two years later, I felt ready to take the advice of my gynecologist. She'd firmly suggested that I eliminate any future risk of cancer by having this surgery. My choice made sense to me now as I recalled her words. "It's just a few snips laparoscopically. Don't worry," she said. "You'll be fine in a few days."

Suddenly, back in the restaurant, I felt the warmth of Paul's arm on my shoulder. I lifted the lid of the tiny jewel box my mother had given me. There lay a miniature Fabergé egg dangling from a gold chain. It was delicate but solid, the color of an ivory tusk with an eggshell-blue band and little sparkles around it. It was a symbol of the steadfast love and life I've received time and again despite heavy loss. I sobbed into my salad and thanked everyone for their gifts. My heart surged with gratitude.

I worked out my true feelings that same night in my journal:

> *With heartache, Paul and I have accepted the fact of our not having children. We'd let go (most of the time) of the desire to be parents and raise a child of our own, but the removal of my ovaries is so final—the last thread of fertility. I feel old. My head knows I'm choosing life again with this decision, but my heart wonders at the taking away of more "womanly parts," as Grammie calls them. Will my skin crinkle too fast and my heart mourn too long?*
>
> *—April 2005*

After the party, I wore my necklace every day, even to the surgery. I tucked it into my pants pocket for safekeeping. It would be there for me after I woke up. I wear it as a reminder to honor myself—inside and out.

Called to Rise

I stood on the podium at the American Cancer Society's Relay for Life. I'd been chosen to share my story and to say something inspiring before the spring rain turned the fields into flood plains. I hated cancer fundraisers, especially ones like these where everyone's crying over someone who died and coming up to you to see if you're still alive. But this day was different. I had a lot to say about where I'd been and how I'd climbed the mountain of recovery to the top.

I scanned the crowd of red, green, and white umbrellas with cancer survivors standing underneath them in their purple T-shirts. It was drizzling lightly, but the clouds dried up momentarily before I went on. Paul, like me, wore the trademark purple shirt given to all who registered as survivors. When we first arrived, I bribed Paul into wearing the shirt over his jeans. It was the first out-in-public cancer event we had ever done together. His hand was sweaty in mine as he walked me to the stage and gave me a good luck kiss.

> *I felt naked up there. Telling my story to five hundred people was a new milestone for me. With a quivering voice, I quoted my favorite poet Emily D. about rising high:*
>   We never know how high we are,
>   till we are called to rise
>   And then, if we are true to plan
>   our statures touch the skies.
>   —*June 2006*

I thanked my parents, my support-group buddies, my friends. Paul hung in the back with my folks, my brother David, and our friends,

Peter and Tina. I thanked the hospital, my doctors and nurses, and the whole community of healing who helped me through the past decade. The microphone grew more comfortable in my hand and my voice got stronger as my litany continued. I thanked the friends I'd known whose spirit was still present despite their passing on to someplace else.

I spoke into the eyes of a bald woman named Ellen, wheeled up front by her husband. Ellen had just completed treatment for brain cancer. She was paralyzed, hunched over, and unable to walk but there, listening to me. She wore a purple shirt too. I spoke to her about what I knew about hope and how we carried it for each other. That's the secret of survivorship, I said. That's the relay gift. Some days, I'd need it. On others, I'd hold it for you like the umbrella clutched in your watchful partner's hand. Applause covered me like a soft rain, and I hopped off the stage with a smile, joining Paul and the other survivors on the track. We marched along with my family for several laps and then aimed for our car. By then, I wanted to run home and get on with the rest of my life, far away from the Ellens and others who weren't doing so well who reminded me of where the wild things are.

My relay speech came back to me a few weeks later as I sat in the emergency room waiting for an X-ray. My collarbone was hurting, hurtling me back five years to that terrifying moment when cancer snuck back into my body and fractured my bone. Determined to mine the dust bunnies under the sagging sofa, I'd reached in too far, heard a crack, and felt an icy fear surge through me again. That crunching bone-on-bone pain as I vacuumed the living room floor reminded me how fragile my remission was.

After more tests, I was fit for a figure-eight brace that resembled the uncomfortable twenty-four-hour bra once modeled on TV. Luckily, there wasn't any cancer in my collarbone this time, only another fracture, a *non-union*, the experts called it. Maybe it would heal; maybe it wouldn't. But there was no sign of cancer.

I remembered what Paul told me about mountaintops. A former rock climber, Paul often said things that made sense to me later on. "The mountain is the moment," he reminded me. "There's always going to be another summit to climb and something else around the next bend to deal with." *As in another surprise rock face—a radiated bone that won't heal,* I thought.

The Face of Healing

The other day, our neighbor Lucy called and asked for a favor. Could Paul come over and help shave Andrew's head on Saturday? "I don't want to do it alone," she told me. At two and a half, a haircut was not in little Andrew's plans. Neither was leukemia. Now, the brown, luscious curls on his head and eyelashes were falling out in clumps, a side effect of his chemotherapy.

In preparation, Paul cleaned his shaving gear, comb, and scissors in buckets of rubbing alcohol. In a soft voice, Paul told me he might shave his head first to make it easier on Andrew. I hugged Paul with tears in my eyes. The last time I'd seen Paul bald, he didn't have a hair on his head. We've had a lot of hairdos in our seven married years together and a lot of taking turns for one another.

This time for Paul was a choice. The change lit his face up with kindness. The prospect of doing some small thing to make Lucy's nightmare a little easier quickened each of our steps.

We packed up our mini-salon along with some toys, packets of hot chocolate, and oatmeal cookies. Andrew and Lucy, a single mom by night and nurse by day, live in a tiny yellow dollhouse on the corner of our road. We walked quietly through their backyard and knocked at the storm door. I saw a blue bed sheet covering a kitchen chair through the window.

Like many two-year-olds, Andrew was obsessed with Thomas the Tank Engine. You had to be careful where you walked in their family room or you'd land on your face in some miniature engine room with wooden train tracks set up like Grand Central Station. The cramped room was crowded with the Thomas collection and the video played nonstop on their small television set. I sat down in the middle of

Andrew's tracks and gushed over his new red plastic train connector. Paul watched while I pushed a long trail of trains over a fancy bridge.

"Does Thomas need a haircut too?" I asked.

Andrew's round, pale moon face looked up at me with a scowl as he burrowed his head into Lucy's chest. Some of the medication he was on made his face puffy and his belly as bloated as a Buddha's. When he turned around, you could see the growing bald circle on his head. He no longer resembled the Andrew we knew who'd jump on his kiddie-jeep to visit us and bang on our piano.

With a nod from Lucy, Paul took a seat in the prepped barber's chair and I turned on the electric shaver. BZZZZZZZZZZZ. Paul's silvery silken locks buzzed off easily in my shaking hands. After a few strokes (there wasn't much there to start with), I handed the clippers over to Paul along with a kiss. His scalp was now prickly in some spots and smooth in others.

"Look, Andrew, Paul's finished," Lucy chirped in a too-high voice. "Now it's your turn."

"NO!" he yelled with a croak, as she positioned him on her lap.

For the next few minutes, while Paul sweated and shaved, I distracted Andrew with as many train noises and "Wheels on the Bus" verses as I could recall. Andrew cried all the more until Lucy bribed him with a new steam engine. All was quiet for a second as Paul turned off the shears.

> *Seeing Andrew's bare head today, I flashed on the moment years before when I watched Paul emerge from the barbershop into the chilly March afternoon. Without a beard or strand of hair on his scalp, Paul looked like a Holocaust survivor to me then. That season of illness was yet another long mountain we'd climbed together.*
>
> *—January 2007*

Andrew bellowing, "I want pizza now!" brought me back into Lucy's warm pine kitchen, into the now where we were the helpers—not the patients. Lucy had a gift card from another neighbor and invited us to stay for lunch. I shooed the bald guys and Lucy out the door to pick up the pizza while I cleaned up. With quiet tears, I swept Paul's and Andrew's locks into a small pile and stepped out onto the back porch. Breathing in the sweet morning that was all around me, I saw a new view from the summit, and it was home.

Blossoms

I'm tapping away on my laptop in a freshly painted wicker chair, while Paul bangs away in his backyard woodshop. He's building me a potting bench, today's gift. When I arrived home from school, Paul said he had a surprise for me. One by one, he unloaded clay pots of varying sizes from his truck and placed them at my feet. To the growing stockpile, he added a pair of red gardening clogs, four hanging baskets, two bags of potting soil, and a picture book about using color as a healing medium in the garden. Bloom where you are planted comes to mind. We are doing just that.

> *The art of living well is a delicate balance—easy to manage with the backdrop of humming songbirds and Paul's buzz saw. But on days when I'm stressed with school meetings, unwritten reports, and sessions with kids, I lose that sense of well-being. It spills out all over the place like a hastily grabbed cup of coffee.*
> —*April 2007*

Time and time again, I've had to regain my equilibrium. Listening to my body helps me to pace my energies and pull back when I lose my footing. At times, I've needed to say "no" even when it has meant *undoing* a prior commitment. This rhythm of *doing and undoing* has gotten me into hot water more than once. I've lost a client, ticked off a friend, and called in sick in exchange for a mental health day, but making choices for my health has also been a life-saving tool in my coping repertoire. Creating space, whether in my garden or in my schedule, offers me flexibility and deeper healing.

Along the way, I've gathered other secrets to keep my planter's pot from getting too empty or too full. Weekly individual therapy sessions have helped me to read my inner compass and live with the uncertainty of the cancer journey. The secrets of survivorship are many, and on any given day, I may need them all—or none.

One way to foster this flexibility has been to adjust my workload. After my recurrence, I chose a part-time position with health benefits in a neighboring school district. Reducing my hours from full-time to part-time has been a financial sacrifice. But by allowing my Monday and Friday schedule to be lighter, I've given myself more time for the other things that support my wellness. Whether it's Friday morning yoga, journaling at my writing desk, or walking on the beach with a friend on the spur of the moment, these spaces have been crucial to my continued health. With the phrase, "No, I couldn't possibly," waiting in the wings for the right moment, less is more.

Recurrence is a sisterhood no one elects to join. Yet, joining a support group was one of the best recommendations I followed. We listened intently to one another's news—of the courage it took to wear a little black dress with a plunging neckline and managing the often dueling needs of family and work—and we mourned the death of a friend together. Our common ground was cancer, but our circle was about much more than that. We became role models for one another and found ways to move on with grace. I discovered that no one needs to make this journey alone.

> *As I write this now, the sacred circle of women that I've been a member of for over five years has come to a natural end. We're all moving on in different ways with our lives. I no longer feel the need to attend our weekly meeting and look forward to having my Thursday evenings free. There's survivorship in that!*
>
> *Life goes on as does my appointment list. I'm still on cancer watch. I saw my oncologist last week for my quarterly checkup. He started me on a new, stronger medication to protect my bones from recurrence. It has side effects to the kidneys so I need to be monitored closely. My right collarbone hasn't healed and*

continues to worry me. I'm scheduled for an MRI of my neck and chest next month to make sure there is no cancer cropping up. So far so good.
—*May 2007*

Physical limitations continue to be part of my story. My arm and hand swell with lymphedema, a chronic condition and side effect of my mastectomy. I still go twice a month for physical therapy. I've just stumbled upon a fellow cancer survivor on the Web who designs classy compression sleeves and gloves for *lymphedivas* like me. I'm trying to enlist my insurance company in paying for a stylish arm sleeve in shimmering black. In the meantime, after brushing my teeth each morning, I put the bulky nylons on my right arm. These body changes are inconvenient on some days and reminders on others to take care of myself. I've returned to my yoga practice, but heavy lifting, vacuuming, and digging for gold in the garden are out.

This summer, I'll turn forty-five. I carry within my body the lessons, losses, and scars of ten years of cancer survivorship, six of those post recurrence. I've lost a breast, bought an inflatable one, and waved good-bye to my ovaries. My collarbone is perpetually broken, and I just found out I'm walking around with a couple of ribs with hairline fractures. I am a marked woman. All that aside, I feel good. There are days when cancer is still a raw deal. But as I look at my lopsided self in the mirror, oddly enough, I feel *whole*. Cancer is no longer the only lens through which I see the world. *There is so much more to see.*

My life is not what I had planned. It's not the life story I would have chosen, but it's the one I've grown to love—and write about. I had envisioned having a family with Paul, being a mother to our children, chasing kids around the yard. The loss of my ability to have children is one I continue to struggle with on some days. I had not anticipated marrying a man who would battle cancer too. Nor did I ever imagine cancer would return for a third time. But along with these sorrows is the knowledge that my path is blessed with abundance. Paul and I are a family.

It's summer vacation again. We're packing my hot red Mazda for a road trip to Ottawa. I've made new friends through my writing, and we're going to visit them. Peering over a bountiful pot of daisies on my new potting bench, I know mine is a full and joyous life.

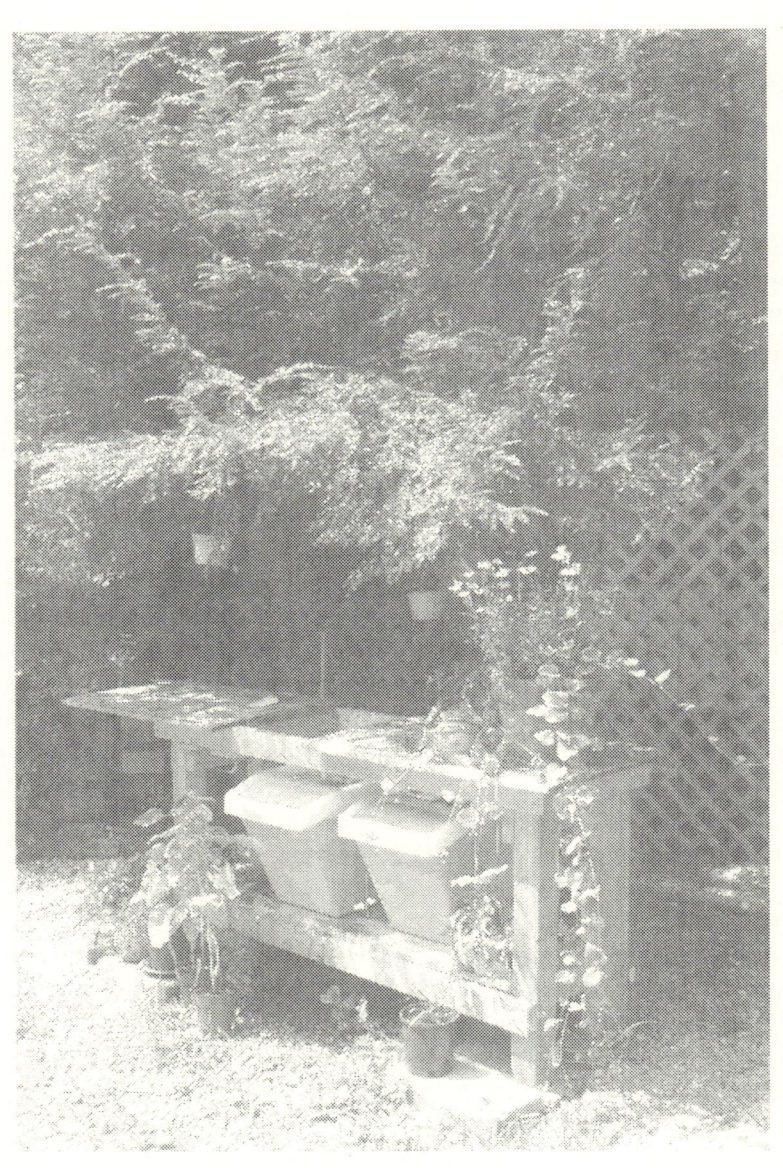

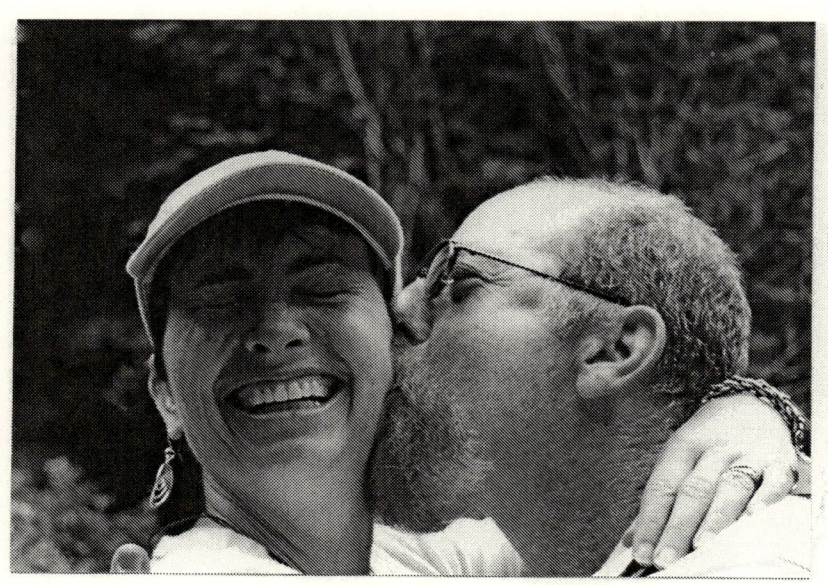

978-0-595-42655-3
0-595-42655-7

Printed in the United States
202152BV00002B/1-240/A